EHRLICHIOSIS

Current Topics in Veterinary Medicine and Animal Science

Volume 54

Ehrlichiosis

A vector-borne disease of animals and humans

Edited by

JIM C. WILLIAMS, Ph.D.

Office of the Director of Intramural Research Programs,
National Institute of Allergy and Infectious Diseases,
Bethesda, Maryland
and
United States Army Medical Research Institute
of Infectious Diseases, Bacteriology Division,
Department of Intracellular Pathogens,
Fort Detrick, Frederick, Maryland, U.S.A.

and

IBULAIMU KAKOMA, D.V.M., Ph.D.

Department of Veterinary Pathobiology and Clinical Medicine,
College of Veterinary Medicine,
University of Illinois,
Urbana, Illinois, U.S.A.

KLUWER ACADEMIC PUBLISHERS

DORDRECHT / BOSTON/ LONDON

Library of Congress Cataloging in Publication Data

Ehrlichiosis : a vector-borne disease of animals and humans / edited
by Jim C. Williams and Ibulaimu Kakoma.
p. cm. -- (Current topics in veterinary medicine and animal
science ; 54)
Based on a symposium held in December 1988 in Washington, DC,
honoring Professor Miodrag Ristic; sponsored by the National
Institute of Allergy and Infectious Diseases and others.
1. Ehrlichiosis--Congresses. 2. Ehrlichia--Congresses.
I. Williams, Jim C. II. Kakoma, Ibulaimu. III. Ristic, Miodrag,
1918- . IV. National Institute of Allergy and Infectious Diseases
(U.S.)
[DNLM: 1. Rickettsiaceae--congresses. 2. Rickettsiaceae
Infections--veterinary--congresses. W1 CU822B v. 54 / SF 809.R5
E33 1988]
QR201.E45E37 1990
636.089'6922--dc20
DNLM/DLC
for Library of Congress 90-4201

ISBN-13: 978-94-010-7394-3 e-ISBN-13: 978-94-009-1998-3
DOI: 10.1007/978-94-009-1998-3

Published by Kluwer Academic Publishers,
P.O. Box 17, 3300 AA Dordrecht, The Netherlands.

Kluwer Academic Publishers incorporates
the publishing programmes of
D. Reidel, Martinus Nijhoff, Dr W. Junk and MTP Press.

Sold and distributed in the U.S.A. and Canada
by Kluwer Academic Publishers,
101 Philip Drive, Norwell, MA 02061, U.S.A.

In all other countries, sold and distributed
by Kluwer Academic Publishers Group,
P.O. Box 322, 3300 AH Dordrecht, The Netherlands.

Printed on acid-free paper

Table of Contents

Preface vii

Acknowledgements ix

List of Contributors xi

CH. 1. The historical background and global importance of ehrlichiosis
D.L. HUXSOLL 1

CH. 2. Current status of the *in-vitro* cultivation of ehrlichiae
M. NYINDO, C.J. HOLLAND, I. KAKOMA 9

CH. 3. Ultrastructure of rickettsiae with special emphasis on ehrlichiae
Y. RIKIHISA 22

CH. 4. Antigenic properties of the ehrlichiae and other rickettsiaceae
G.A. DASCH, E. WEISS, J.C. WILLIAMS 32

CH. 5. Biological properties of the genus *Ehrlichia*: substrate utilization and energy metabolism
E. WEISS, G.A. DASCH, J.C. WILLIAMS, Y-H. KANG 59

CH. 6. Biologic and pathogenic properties of *Ehrlichia risticii*: the etiologic agent of equine monocytic ehrlichiosis
C.J. HOLLAND 68

CH. 7. Pathophysiology of canine ehrlichiosis
I. ABEYGUNAWARDENA, I. KAKOMA, R.D. SMITH 78

CH. 8. Experimental ehrlichiosis in nonhuman primates
E.H. STEPHENSON 93

CH. 9. Human ehrlichiosis in the United States
D.B. FISHBEIN 100

CH. 10. Evolutionary history of chlamydiae: answers for some old questions, no answers for some new ones
J.W. MOULDER 112

CH. 11. Recent research findings on cowdriosis
J.D. BEZUIDENHOUT 125

CH. 12. Current strategies in research on ehrlichiosis
M. RISTIC 136

CH. 13. Epilogue
J.C. WILLIAMS, I. KAKOMA 154

Index of Subjects 159

Preface

This book is a direct result of a symposium held in December 1988, in Washington, DC, honoring Professor Emeritus Miodrag Ristic for his contributions to rickettsial disease research, in general, and, to ehrlichiosis, in particular. He and his colleagues in the United States Army Medical Research Unit brought to the world's attention an epidemic of ehrlichiosis, that occurred in German shepherd dogs during the Vietnam War. The group was able to culture the microorganism *Ehrlichia canis* and to fulfill Koch's postulates. They eventually developed an indirect immunofluorescent antibody (IFA) test which has been adopted internationally. The same group joined a national effort to decipher another mysterious disease known as Potomac horse fever (PHF). They used the same technology developed by Nyindo in Dr. Ristic's laboratory to isolate, characterize, and again develop a similar IFA test for PHF. Today PHF has been diagnosed, at least serologically, practically across the entire United States, in some provinces of Canada, and reports are beginning to trickle in of its occurrence in European countries. Thus, the etiologic agent of PHF, now named after Professor Ristic, *Ehrlichia risticii*, historically places this scientist side by side with the other 2 "R's", i.e., Ricketts and da Rochalima.

Ehrlichiosis is not limited to domestic animals. *Sennetsu rickettsiosis*, long known by Japanese scientists as an imitator of "infectious mononucleosis," was subsequently shown to be caused by an ehrlichial agent, through collaborative efforts among the United States Army, the University of Illinois, and Dr. Tachibana's Laboratory in Japan. More recently, human cases of an *Ehrlichiosis-like syndrome*, confusable, but distinct from Rocky Mountain spotted fever (without a rash) were diagnosed and strongly associated with a history of tick bites. Ehrlichia-like inclusions in mononuclear cells have been demonstrated by workers at the Centers for Disease Control in Atlanta, Georgia, in collaboration with Professor Ristic. The high "heterologous" antibody titer to *Ehrlichia canis* has encouraged scientists to suggest that the putative agent is *E. canis*, but more data beyond serology will be needed to support this hypothesis. Although an ehrlichia-like bacterium has been implicated as the etiologic agent of human disease, we caution the reader that, at this stage, no definitive etiologic proof exists, as no ehrlichia has actually been isolated from these patients.

This publication is not limited to ehrlichiae, but includes some data on all six antigenically distinct groups of rickettsiae pathogenic for humans and animals, i.e., *Rickettsia typhi, R. rickettsii, R. tsutsugamushi, Coxiella burnetii, Rochalimaea quintana*, and *Ehrlichia* species, as well as observations on recent findings on Chlamydiae and *Cowdria ruminantium*. The ehrlichiae are leukocytic rickettsiae with a preference for growth in the phagosome of either monocytic or granulocytic cells.

The successful adaptation of *in-vitro* methods of propagation of various ehrlichiae and rickettsiae has facilitated a number of biochemical, immunologic, immunodiagnostic, genetic and molecular biology studies on these obligate intracellular bacteria. In the near future, more diagnostic techniques, e.g. DNA and/or RNA-based probes, will be developed. Such tools will enhance our knowledge of the taxonomy of these agents and perhaps lead to the identification of hitherto unrecognized rickettsial pathogens of humans and animals.

The papers presented at the December 1988 symposium were revised on the basis of more recent work in 1989.

J. C. Williams, Ph.D.
I. Kakoma, D.V.M., Ph.D.
editors

Acknowledgements

We are grateful to our sponsors, the National Institute of Allergy and Infectious Diseases, Bethesda, Maryland; Rhone Merieux, Lyon, France; Norden Laboratories, Lincoln, Nebraska; Kirkegaard and Perry Laboratories, Gaithersburg, Maryland; Pitman-Moore, Terre Haute, Indiana; and Integrated Diagnostics, Inc., Baltimore, Maryland. We are indebted to the American Society of Tropical Medicine and Hygiene, and the American Society of Tropical Veterinary Medicine Scientific Program Committees for support in organizing the symposium.

We are also indebted to Ms. N. Dekker and Ms. A. D. E. Greeven of Kluwer Academic Publishers for their patience and advice; to Ms. Betty Martin; and Ms. Marilyn Lynch for their patient preparation of this volume, and to Dr. D. L. Huxsoll, Dr. E. Weiss, Dr. D. M. Waag, and Ms. K. Kenyon for carefully reading this volume.

List of Contributors

ABEYGUNAWARDENA, I, College of Veterinary Medicine, University of Peredeniya, Peredeniya, Sri Lanka.

BEZUIDENHOUT, JD, Veterinary Research Institute, Onderstepoort, 0110, Republic of South Africa

DASCH, GA, Rickettsial Disease Division, Naval Medical Research Institute, Bethesda, Maryland 20814-5055, USA

FISHBEIN, DB, Viral and Rickettsial Zoonoses Branch, Division of Viral and Rickettsial Diseases, Center for Infectious Diseases, Centers for Disease Control, United States Public Health Service, Atlanta, Georgia 30333, USA

HOLLAND, CJ, University of Illinois, College of Veterinary Medicine, Department of Veterinary Pathobiology, Urbana, Illinois 61801, USA

HUXSOLL, DL, Commander, United States Army Medical Research Institute of Infectious Diseases, Fort Detrick, Frederick, Maryland 21701-5011, USA

KAKOMA, I, Departments of Veterinary Pathobiology and Clinical Medicine, College of Veterinary Medicine, University of Illinois, Urbana, Illinois 61801, USA

KANG, Y-H, Department of Pathology, Naval Medical Research Institute, Bethesda, Maryland 20814, USA

MOULDER, JW, Deparment of Molecular Genetics and Cell Biology, The University of Chicago, Chicago, Illinois 60637, USA: Present address, 10349 East Edna Place, Tucson, Arizona 85748, USA

NYINDO, M, International Center for Insect Physiology and Ecology (ICIPE), P. O. Box 30772, Nairobi, Kenya

RIKIHISA, Y, Department of Veterinary Pathobiology, College of Veterinary Medicine, The Ohio State University, Columbus, Ohio 43210-1092, USA

RISTIC, M, Department of Veterinary Pathobiology, College of Veterinary Medicine, University of Illinois, Urbana, Illinois 61801, USA

SMITH, RD, University of Illinois, Department of Veterinary Pathobiology, Urbana, Illinois 61801, USA

STEPHENSON, ED, Virginia-Maryland Regional College of Veterinary Medicine, The University of Maryland, College Park, Maryland 20742, USA

WEISS, E, Rickettsial Diseases Division, Naval Medical Research Institute, Bethesda, Maryland 20814-5055, USA

WILLIAMS JC, Office of the Director of Intramural Research Programs, National Institute of Allergy and Infectious Diseases, Bethesda, Maryland 20892; United States Army Medical Research Institute of Infectious Diseases, Bacteriology Division Department of Intracellular Pathogens, Fort Detrick, Frederick, Maryland 21701-5011, USA

1. THE HISTORICAL BACKGROUND AND GLOBAL IMPORTANCE OF EHRLICHIOSIS

DAVID L. HUXSOLL, D.V.M., Ph.D.

Abstract

Ehrlichiosis is caused by a group of small, pleomorphic microorganisms found in circulating leukocytes of susceptible mammalian hosts. The tribe Ehlichiae, which includes a number of species infecting animals, is a member of the family Rickettsiaceae. In the 1984 edition of Bergey's Manual, *Rickettsia sennetsu*, the etiologic agent of human "sennetsu rickettsiosis" in western Japan, was moved to the genus *Ehrlichia*, based on morphological, cultural, and antigenic characteristics. For the first time, the genus *Ehrlichia* included a species causing human disease. The recent identification of an ehrlichial agent, *E. risticii*, as the cause of Potomac horse fever (PHF) is evidence of the importance of this group of microorganisms as the cause of disease in animals. More recently, ehrlichial infections have been implicated in humans with disease that appears to be similar to Rocky Mountain spotted fever (RMSF). The diagnosis was based on morphological characteristics of infected leukocytes and serological studies, which served to suggest that the infecting microorganism is closely related to *Ehrlichia canis*.

Ehrlichiosis, an Emerging Problem for Humans and Animals

Ehrlichial diseases that have emerged as significant problems for humans and animals over the past two decades include some old acquaintances and some that are new with respect to identity and concept. Ehrlichiosis is caused by small, pleomorphic, obligate intracellular bacteria which parasitize the cytoplasmic phagosomes of mononuclear or polymorphonuclear leukocytes. The bacteria are members of the genus *Ehrlichia*, tribe Ehrlichiae, family Rickettsiaceae, and are often observed in compact colonies or phagosomal inclusions (morulae). As all rickettsiologists are aware, the amount of work on their favorite subject over time has been marked by peaks and valleys that seem to exceed those of other major classes of infectious microorganisms. Work on rickettsial diseases has often peaked in response to an urgent need, such as a military operation, when the disease threatened the outcome of a campaign or even a war. Examples are epidemic typhus, etiologic agent *Rickettsia prowazekii*, and scrub typhus, etiologic agent *R. tsutsugamushi*, during and after World War II. In assessing the significant findings, observations, and milestones in research on ehrlichiosis that have enabled us to get where we are today, we again go back to a wartime situation, namely United States military action in Southeast Asia in the 1960s.

J. C. Williams and I. Kakoma (eds.), Ehrlichiosis, 1–8.

Although *E. canis*, the type species of the genus *Ehrlichia*, was discovered by Donatien and Lestoquard in 1935 [10], it was not until 1967, when an outbreak of disease in military working dogs in Vietnam showed the full pathogenic potential of *E. canis* [21, 33]. The disease that became known as tropical canine pancytopenia (TCP) was clinically distinct from any disease previously described and eventually accounted for the death of 200-300 military dogs [26]. In order to control the disease, a major research strategy was launched, involving both military and university laboratories, which led to means for controlling the disease, and to a greater understanding of ehrlichial agents. Many subsequent research accomplishments on this important group of disease agents for man and animals would not have been possible had it not been for the early work on *E. canis* after the outbreak of TCP in Southeast Asia (Fig 1).

After the discovery of *E. canis* in tick-infested dogs in Algeria in 1935, the infection was identified in dogs in various parts of Africa, the Middle East, and the Orient [13]. In 1957, Bool and Sutmoller [3] identified *E. canis* in dogs in Aruba, documenting its first recognition in the Western Hemisphere. In the United States, the first case of canine ehrlichiosis was reported by Ewing in 1963 as a *Babesia canis* infection [12]. Prior to the outbreak in military working dogs in Southeast Asia, canine ehrlichiosis was considered to be a relatively mild disease characterized by fever, vomiting, and naso-ocular discharges [13].

The highly fatal form of canine ehrlichiosis in military dogs in Southeast Asia was known as TCP and was characterized by hemorrhage, pancytopenia, and severe debilitation. This form of the disease was observed as early as 1963 in British military dogs in Singapore [34]. In 1967, the disease occurred in several Labrador retrievers trained as tracker dogs, and shipped from a British training center in Malaysia to the United States military in Vietnam. In 1968, an epizootic of the disease occurred in Vietnam among German shepherd dogs that had originated from the United States [33]. Subsequently, it was learned that a similar disease had occurred primarily in German shepherd dogs in the Virgin Islands [21], Puerto Rico [21], and Florida [29]. Concurrent with the identification and confirmation of *E. canis* as the etiologic agent of TCP, the efficacy of tetracycline for prophylaxis and therapy was demonstrated [2, 9].

Extensively documented studies of experimental infections in beagle and German shepherd dogs showed that the severity of TCP is dependent on the breed of dog [20, 22]. Both breeds of dogs were readily infected and they developed acute signs of disease 7 to 10 days after inoculation (Fig. 2). Notably only German shepherd dogs developed the severe chronic disease, usually 2 to 3 months postinoculation, after initial signs of infection had abated [7, 22]. The hemorrhage was associated with severe pancytopenia resulting from bone marrow aplasia [6, 16]. Approximately two thirds of experimentally infected German shepherd dogs developed bone marrow aplasia and hemorrhage. The pancytopenia observed early in the infection could not be attributed to marrow failure. However, a generalized disease of the bone marrow was apparently established during the convalescent period, thereby compromising bone marrow function and inducing the severe chronic disease (Fig. 2).

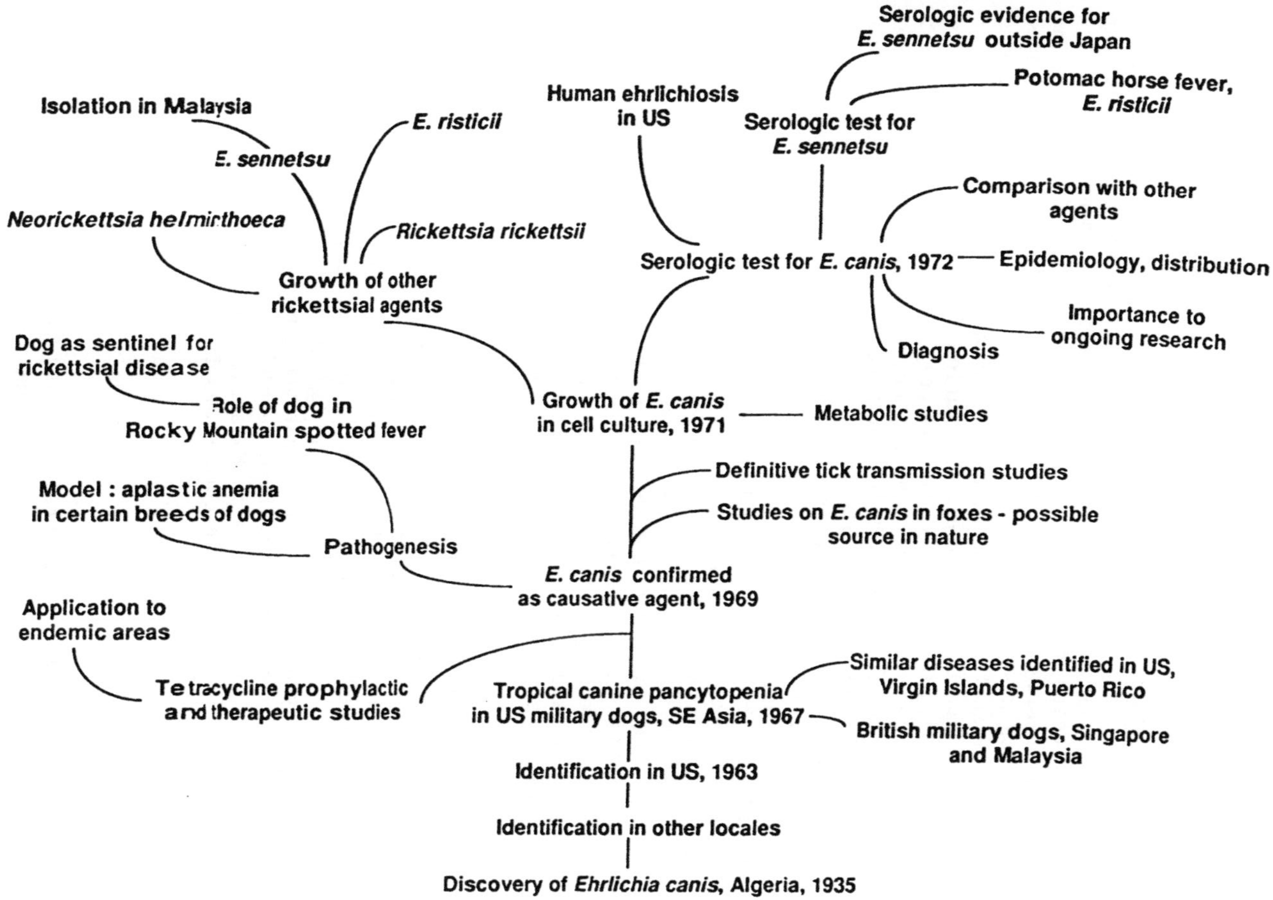

Figure 1. Research stimulated by the outbreak of tropical canine pancytopenia in United States military working dogs in Southeast Asia.

Marrow hypoplasia (e.g., aplastic anemia) may be a result of persistent infection which promotes a failure or suppression of pluripotent myeloid stem cells. The aplastic anemia maybe immunologically mediated by autoimmune destruction of platelets and the marrow microenvironment. These studies established that dogs could become infected for years. Beagle and German shepherd dogs that do not develop bone marrow aplasia and are not treated with tetracycline develop a mild chronic infection without clinical signs and with Ehrlichemia (Fig. 2) [14, 20]. This stage of disease is possibly a carrier state that promotes transmission of ehrlichiae from the dog, to the tick vector and to humans.

Pathogenesis studies of *E. canis* led to experiments with *Rickettsia rickettsii*, the etiologic agent of RMSF, in the dog [25]. The findings showed that the dog was highly susceptible to infection by *R. rickettsii* and developed clinical signs of disease. Studies in Malaysia showed that dogs could be used as sentinels for murine typhus and scrub typhus [23]. Experimental infections in red and gray foxes demonstrated that those species can be readily infected, but develop few signs of disease [1]. These observations have led to the hypothesis that wild canidae may serve as reservoirs for *E. canis*.

In multiple studies with hundreds of ticks, *Rhipicephalus sanguineus* was confirmed as a vector of canine ehrlichiosis [15]. Transstadial transmission was readily demonstrated. Transovarial transmission of *E. canis*, as reported by Donatien and Lestoquard [11], was not confirmed, although many attempts were made.

The accomplishment that undoubtedly had the greatest impact on the study of ehrlichial agents was the propagation of *E. canis* in cell cultures established by Nyindo and coworkers from leukocytes of infected dogs [28]. This *in-vitro* cultivation of *E. canis* allowed the development of a serologic test with infected cells as the *in-situ* antigen [32]. The applications of the serologic tests are depicted in Figure 1. These tests provided much more than a means of diagnosis: research was aided; information on the distribution of *E. canis* was acquired [8, 24], serologic relationships of *E. canis* to *E. sennetsu* and other ehrlichial agents were demonstrated [18, 31], evidence for *E. sennetsu* infections outside of Japan was collected [30], the etiologic agent of PHF was identified as an ehrlichial agent [18], and evidence for human ehrlichiosis in the United States was gathered [27].

The techniques used to grow *E. canis* in cell cultures have been applied to other rickettsiae, including *R. rickettsii* [5] and *Neorickettsia helminthoeca* [4], the causative agent of salmon poisoning in dogs. In a major development after serologic studies that provided evidence of *E. sennetsu* infections in Malaysia, isolations were made of *E. sennetsu* or closely related microorganisms from patients with febrile disease in Malaysia [17, 19].

Summary

Much progress in understanding ehrlichiae and the diseases they cause has been made in the past 20 years. The importance of these obligate intracellular bacteria in the infection of humans and animals is more fully appreciated. There are still many unanswered questions. A cursory

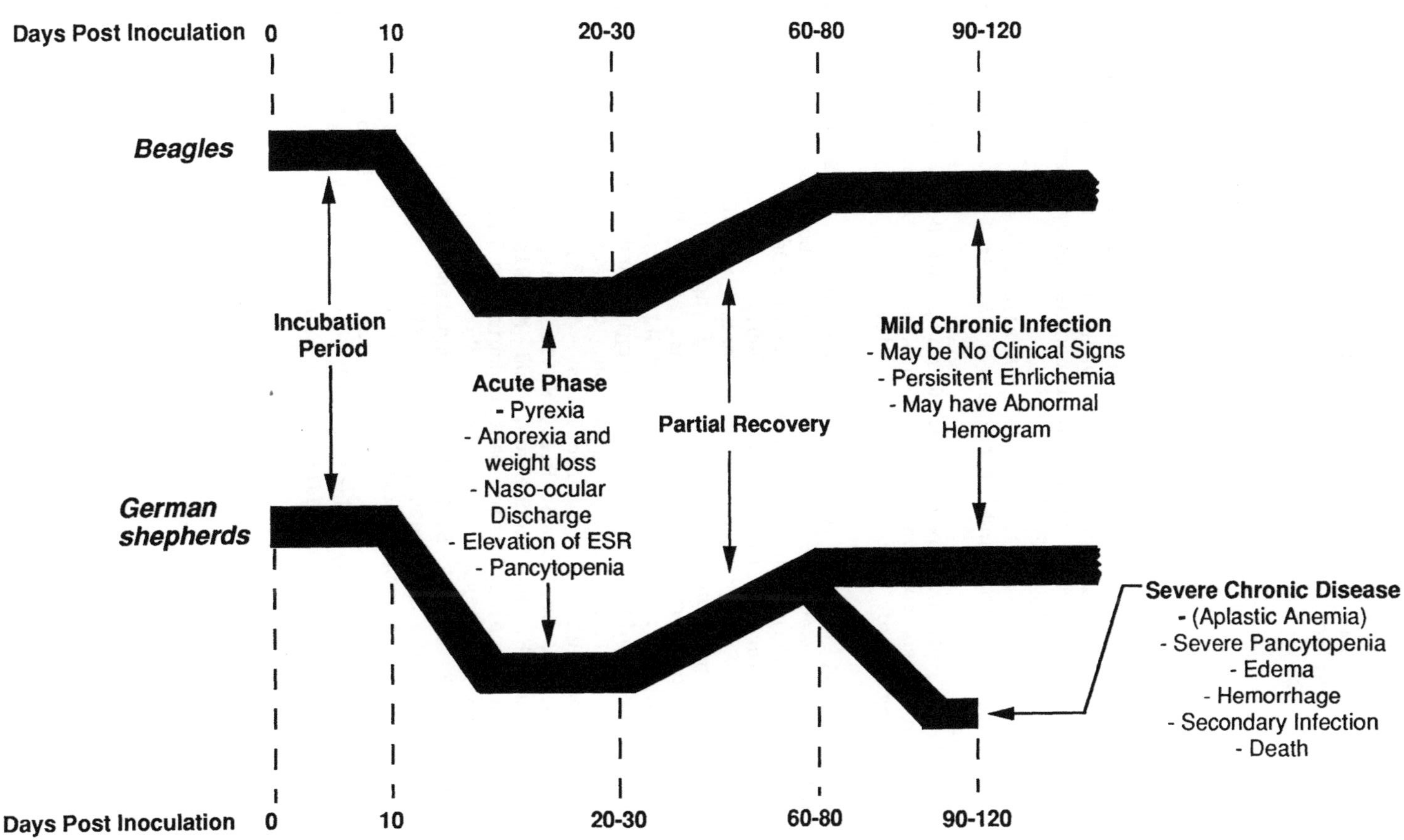

Figure 2. Courses of experimental infection with *Ehrlichia canis* in beagles and German shepherds are similar up to 60 days post-infection.

examination of the chronology of research accomplishments in Figure 1 clearly shows where new research initiatives are needed. Where will the new research initiatives lead in the next 5 to 10 years?

Literature Cited

1. **Amyx, H. L. and D. L. Huxsoll.** 1973. Red and gray foxes - potential reservoir hosts for *Ehrlichia canis*. *J. Wildl. Dis.*. **9**:47-50.
2. **Amyx, H. L., D. L. Huxsoll, D. C. Zeiler, and P. K. Hildebrandt.** 1971. Therapeutic and prophylactic value of tetracycline in dogs infected with the agent of tropical canine pancytopenia. *J. Am. Vet. Med. Assoc.* **159**:1428-1432.
3. **Bool, P. H. and P. Sutmoller.** 1957. *Ehrlichia canis* infections in dogs on Aruba (Netherlands Antilles). *J. Am. Vet. Med. Assoc.* **130**:418-420.
4. **Brown, J. L., D. L. Huxsoll, M. Ristic, and P. K. Hildebrandt.** 1972. In vitro cultivation of *Neorickettsia helminthoeca*, the causative agent of salmon poisoning disease. *Am. J. Vet. Res.* **33**:1695-1700.
5. **Buhles, W. C., Jr., D. L. Huxsoll, and B. L. Elisberg.** 1973. Isolation of *Rickettsia rickettsii* in primary bone marrow cell and circulating monocyte cultures derived from experimentally infected guinea pigs. *Infect. Immun.* **7**:1003-1005.
6. **Buhles, W. C. Jr., D. L. Huxsoll, and P. Hildebrandt.** 1975. Tropical canine pancytopenia: role of aplastic anemia in the pathogenesis of severe disease. *J. Comp. Path.* **85**:511-521.
7. **Buhles, W. C., Jr., D. L. Huxsoll, and M. Ristic.** 1974. Tropical canine pancytopenia: clinical, hematologic, and serologic response of dogs to *Ehrlichia canis* infection, tetracycline therapy, and challenge inoculation. *J. Infect. Dis.* **130**:357-367.
8. **Davidson, D. E., Jr., G. S. Dill, M. Tingpalapong, M. Premabutra, P. L. Nguen, E. H. Stephenson, and M. Ristic.** 1975 Canine ehrlichiosis (tropical canine pancytopenia) in Thailand. *Southeast Asian J. Trop. Med. Pub. Hlth.* **Vol 6:** No. 4.
9. **Davidson, D. E. Jr., G. S. Dill, M. Tingpalapong, M. Premabutra, P. L. Nugen, E. H. Stephenson, and M. Ristic.** Prophylactic and therapeutic use of tetracycline during an epizootic of ehrlichiosis among military dogs. *J. Am. Vet. Med. Assoc.* **172:** No. 6:697-699.
10. **Donatien, A. and F. Lestoquard.** 1935. Existence en Algérie d'une Ricketttsia du chien. *Bulletin de la Societé* de Pathologie Exotique. **28**:418-419.
11. **Donatien, A. and F. Lestoquard.** 1937. État actuel des connaissances sur les Rickettsioses animales. *Archives de l'Institut Pasteur d'Algé*rie. **15**:142-187.
12. **Ewing, S. A.** 1963. Observations on leukocytic inclusion bodies from dogs infected with *Babesia canis*. *J. Am. Vet. Med. Assoc.* **143**:503-506.
13. **Ewing, S. A.** 1969. Canine ehrlichiosis. *Adv. Vet. Comp. Med.* **13**:331-353.

14. **Ewing, S. A. and R. G. Buckner.** 1965. Observations on the incubation period and persistence of *Ehrlichia* species in experimentally infected dogs. *Vet. Med./Sm. Ann. Clin.* **60**:152-155.
15. **Groves, M. G., G. L. Dennis, H. L. Amyx, and D. L. Huxsoll.** 1975. Transmission of *Ehrlichia canis* to dogs by *Rhipicephalus sanguineus* ticks. *Am. J. Vet. Res.* **36**:937-940.
16. **Hildebrandt, P. K., D. L. Huxsoll, J. S. Walker, R. M. Nims, R. Taylor, and M. Andrews.** 1973. Pathology of canine ehrlichiosis (tropical canine pancytopenia). *Am. J. Vet. Res.* **34**:1309-1320.
17. **Hoilien, C. A., M. Ristic, D. L. Huxsoll, and G. Rapmund.** 1982. *Rickettsia sennetsu* in human blood monocyte cultures: similarities to the growth cycle of *Ehrlichia canis*. *Infect. Immun.* **35**:314-319.
18. **Holland, C. J., M. Ristic, A. I. Cole, P. Johnson, G. Baker, and T. Goetz.** 1985. Isolation, experimental transmission and characterization of causative agent of Potomac horse fever. *Science* **227**:522-524.
19. **Holland, C. J., M. Ristic, D. L. Huxsoll, A. I. Cole, and G. Rapmund.** 1985. Adaption of *Ehrlichia sennetsu* to canine blood monocytes: preliminary structural and serological studies with cell culture-derived *Ehrlichia sennetsu*. *Infect. Immun.* 366-371.
20. **Huxsoll, D. L.** 1976. Canine ehrlichiosis (tropical canine pancytopenia): a review, *In* Veterinary Parasitology, Elsevier Sci. Pub. Co., Amsterdam. **2**:49-60.
21. **Huxsoll, D. L., P. K. Hildebrandt, R. M. Nims, J. A. Fergurson, and J. S. Walker.** 1969. *Ehrlichia canis* - the causative agent of a hemorrhagic disease of dogs? *Vet. Rec.* **85**:587.
22. **Huxsoll, D. L., P. K. Hildebrandt, R. M. Nims, and J. S. Walker.** 1970. Tropical canine pancytopenia. *J. Am. Vet. Med. Assoc.* **157**:1627-1632.
23. **Huxsoll, D. L., A. Shirai, D. M. Robinson, L. F. Yap, and B. L. Lim.** 1977. Presence of antibodies to scrub typhus and murine typhus in dogs from Selangor, Peninsular Malaysia. *Southeast Asian J. Trop. Med. Pub. Hlth.* **8**: No. 2.
24. **Keefe, T. J., C. J. Holland, P. E. Salyer, and M. Ristic.** 1982. Distribution of *Ehrlichia canis* among military working dogs in the world and selected civilian dogs in the United States. *J. Am. Vet. Med. Assoc.* **181**:236-238.
25. **Keenan, K. P., W. C. Buhles, D. L. Huxsoll, R. G. Williams, and P. K. Hildebrandt.** 1977. Studies on the pathogenesis of *Rickettsia rickettsii* in the dog: clinical and clinicopathologic changes of experimental infection. *Am. J. Vet. Res.* **38**:No. 6, 851-856.
26. **Kelch, W. J.** 1984. The canine ehrlichiosis (tropical canine pancytopenia) epizootic in Vietnam and its implications for the veterinary care of military working dogs. *Milit. Med.* **149**:327-331.
27. **Maeda K., N. Markowitz, R. C. Hawley, M. Ristic, D. Cox, and J. McDade.** 1987. Human infection with *Ehrlichia canis*, a leukocytic rickettsia. *N. Eng. J. Med.* **316**:853-856.

28. **Nyindo, M. B. A., M. Ristic, D. L. Huxsoll, and A. R. Smith.** 1971. Tropical canine pancytopenia: in vitro cultivation of the causative agent, *Ehrlichia canis*. *Am. J. Vet. Res.* **32**:1651-1658.
29. **Ridout, S.** 1969. Eau Gollie, FL. Personal communication.
30. **Ristic, M.** 1986. Pertinent characteristics of leukocytic rickettsiae of humans and animals, pp. 182-187, *In* L. Leive (ed.), Microbiology -- 1986. American Society for Microbiology, Washington D.C.
31. **Ristic, M., D. L. Huxsoll, N. Tachibana, and G. Rapmund.** 1981. Evidence of a serologic relationship between *Ehrlichia canis* and *Rickettsia sennetsu*. *Am. J. Trop. Med. Hyg.* **30**:1324-1328.
32. **Ristic, M., D. L. Huxsoll, R. M. Weisiger, P. K. Hildebrandt, and M. B. A. Nyindo.** 1972. Serological diagnosis of tropical canine pancytopenia by indirect immunofluorescence. *Infect. Immun.* **6**:226-231.
33. **Walker, J. S., J. D. Rundquist, R. Taylor, B. L. Wilson, M. R. Andrews, J. Barck, A. L. Hogge, Jr., D. L. Huxsoll, P. K. Hildebrandt, and R. M. Nims.** 1970. Clinical and clinicopathologic findings in tropical canine pancytopenia. *J. Am. Vet. Med. Assoc.* **157**:43-55.
34. **Wilkins, J. H., R. S. T. Bowden, and G. T. Wilkinson.** 1967. A new canine disease syndrome. *Vet. Rec.* **81**:57-58.

2. CURRENT STATUS OF THE *IN-VITRO* CULTIVATION OF EHRLICHIAE

Mramba Nyindo, D.V.M., Ph.D,
Cynthia J. Holland, Ph.D,
Ibulaimu Kakoma, D.V.M., Ph.D

Abstract

The first successful method for the *in-vitro* propagation of *Ehrlichia canis* nearly 20 years ago facilitated the identification of other members of this genus. Since then, significant progress has been made on the adaptation of techniques for the *in-vitro* cultivation of other leukocytic rickettsiae. Consequently, specific serologic tests e.g., indirect immunofluorescent antibody (IFA), are well established for the surveillance of infections caused by *E. canis, E. sennetsu,* and, more recently, *E. risticii*. In addition, large-scale propagation of these agents has facilitated studies on the pathological, biochemical, and molecular aspects of this group of microorganisms. Techniques developed thus far will enhance our knowledge on the genus *Ehrlichia* and, perhaps, aid in the identification of additional species of *Ehrlichia* affecting humans.

Introduction

Members of the genus *Ehrlichia* are a group of obligate intraphagosomal bacteria of similar morphology which parasitize circulating leukocytes of wild and domestic animals and humans [30]. Although *Ehrlichia canis*, the type species of the genus *Ehrlichia*, was first recognized in 1934 [4], its pathogenic potential for dogs was recognized in 1968. Between 1968 and 1970, a major epidemic of canine ehrlichiosis, a term synonymous with tropical canine pancytopenia (TCP), resulted in the loss of hundreds of military working dogs in Vietnam [13]. Since then, canine ehrlichiosis is recognized throughout the United States and elsewhere [17].

After the severe losses of dogs in Vietnam, an intensive research effort resulted in the first *in-vitro* cultivation of *E. canis* [23] and the subsequent development of a serodiagnostic test procedure [31]. In the last decade, the use of this test as an aid in diagnosis of the disease has served to confirm the presence of canine ehrlichiosis throughout the United States and in many other parts of the world wherever the vector, the brown dog tick, *Rhipicephalus sanguineous*, exists [17].

The advances in the knowledge of the biological properties of *E. canis* has led to the recent recognition of its close relationship with a human pathogen, *Rickettsia sennetsu* [9, 32]. The latter rickettsia is the etiologic agent of sennetsu rickettsiosis, a mononucleosis-like syndrome, which occurs primarily in Japan and other regions of Southeast

J. C. Williams and I. Kakoma (eds.), Ehrlichiosis, 9–21.

Asia. This finding led to the reclassification of *R. sennetsu* as *species incertae sedis* [22] to the genus *Ehrlichia* under the name *Ehrlichia sennetsu* [30]. The similarity between the two agents was further substantiated on the basis of their common morphologic properties and their preference for growth in blood monocytes [8, 9, 11].

In 1984, a new ehrlichial pathogen [10, 29] was discovered as the etiologic agent of equine monocytic ehrlichiosis (EME), commonly known as Potomac horse fever (PHF). Retrospective serological studies have identified PHF as a unique clinical disease affecting horses since 1979 [18]. PHF appears to be endemic throughout the United States and Canada with some cases reported in France and Italy [33]. The rickettsial etiology of PHF was identified when sera obtained from convalescent horses were shown to react strongly against *E. sennetsu* antigen in the IFA test and, to a lesser degree, against *E. canis* [10]. The bacterial agent was then isolated in cultures of peripheral blood monocytes obtained from an experimentally infected pony by techniques previously described for *Ehrlichia* isolation [11, 12, 23]. Subsequently, the newly isolated strain was confirmed to be a unique member of the genus *Ehrlichia*. The isolate was named *Ehrlichia risticii*, in honor of Miodrag Ristic.

Unlike *E. canis, E. sennetsu*, and *E. risticii*, which parasitize blood monocytes, *E. equi* and *E. phagocytophila* primarily invade circulating granulocytes. *Ehrlichia equi* is the etiologic agent of equine ehrlichiosis, whereas *E. phagocytophila* causes tick-borne fever affecting sheep, cattle, and bison [30, 34]. The above two microorganisms are morphologically similar to other members of the genus *Ehrlichia*. Limited studies have, thus far, determined the existence of antigenic relationships between *E. equi, E. canis*, and *E. sennetsu* [32, 34]. Since granulocytes cannot be maintained *in vitro* for more than a few days, and no granulocytic precursor cell lines are available, the continuous *in-vitro* propagation of *E. equi* and *E. phagocytophila* has not been achieved. Hence, the subject matter of this paper will be confined to the monocytic ehrlichiae.

In-Vitro Cultivation of *E. Canis*

Early studies on *E. canis* concentrated on the disease and its transmission, providing little information on the biological properties of the bacterium. This lack of progress was primarily due to inefficient methods for the *in-vitro* propagation of *E. canis*. The microorganism exhibits extreme host specificity, thereby preventing any studies with established cell lines, laboratory animals, or chicken embryos [14, 15, 20]. Because of the severe epizootic of TCP affecting military working dogs in Southeast Asia during the Vietnam era, an urgent need was recognized for the development of control measures. The need for the propagation of the pathogen and a suitable diagnostic test prompted research efforts for devising a method for the *in-vitro* cultivation of the agent. Nyindo et al. [23] were successful in culturing the pathogen in the peripheral blood monocytes obtained from experimentally infected dogs during the acute phase of the disease. The

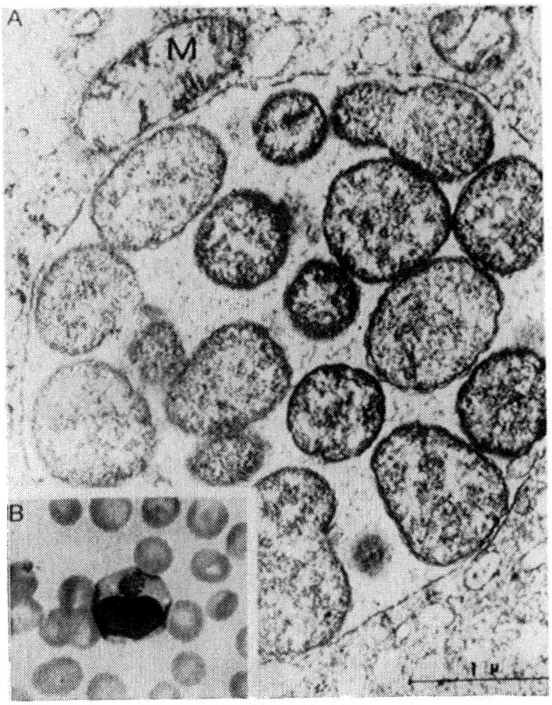

Figure 1. A. Electron micrograph of ***Ehrlichia canis*** inclusion (morula) within the cytoplasm of a cultured canine monocyte. Note that the microorganisms are contained within a cytoplasmic phagosomal vacuole. B. Peripheral blood smear from a dog acutely infected with *E. canis* revealing an *E. canis* inclusion within the cytoplasm of a monocyte. Giemsa stain.

key to this success was the development of the monocyte culture with the exclusion of antibiotics from the medium. Culture medium consisted of Minimum Essential Medium (MEM) supplemented with 1% L-glutamine and 20% heat-inactivated autologous dog serum. This method of cultivation revealed a developmental cycle of *E. canis* which resembled superficially that of the chlamydiae [26]. Microorganisms appeared to replicate in phagosomal vacuoles within the host-cell cytoplasm (Fig. 1) [23]. The initial phase of growth revealed small cells (0.2 to 0.4 μm in diameter) followed by larger cells (0.5 to 4 μm in diameter) within a vacuole. The developing cells filled the mature inclusion (morula) by 12 to 17 days after culture initiation. Some cells contained up to 70 intracytoplasmic morulae (Fig. 2). Antibody specific for *E. canis*, obtained from the serum of a dog during the chronic phase of infection, was

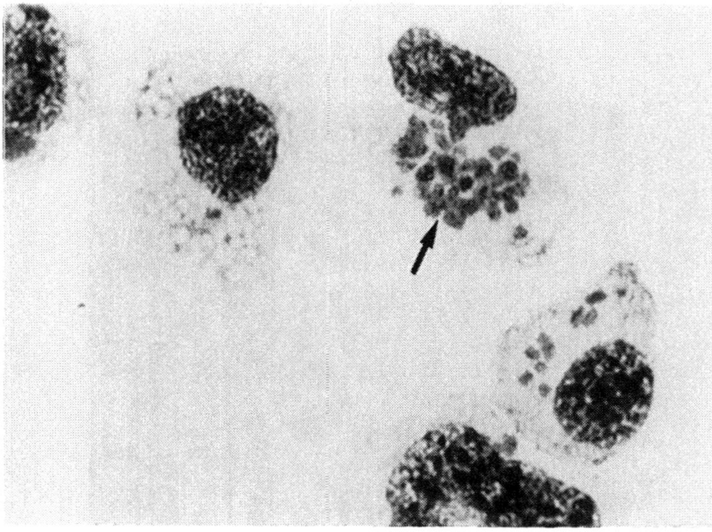

Figure 2. *Ehrlichia canis*-infected peripheral blood monocyte cultures. One cell contains numerous inclusions (arrow). Giemsa stain.

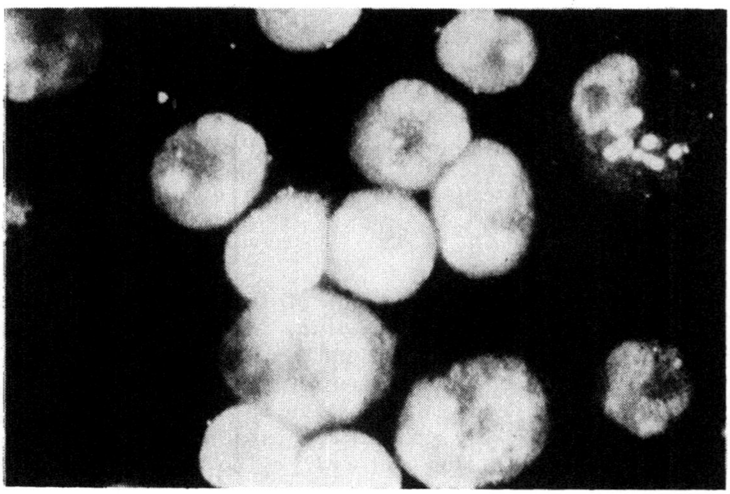

Figure 3. Direct fluorescent antibody test for *Ehrlichia canis* demonstrating specific fluorescence of the cytoplasmic inclusions in cultured canine monocytes.

conjugated with fluorescein isothiocyanate and reacted with antigen obtained from the above cell cultures showing specific fluorescence of the microorganisms within the morulae of the host cell cytoplasm (Fig. 3) [31].

The method of *in-vitro* cultivation was later modified by transferring supernatant fluid containing *E. canis*-infected host cells to normal primary canine monocyte cell cultures obtained from noninfected dogs [6]. This method resulted in successful infection of normal cell cultures, thus, allowing the continuous *in-vitro* propagation of *E. canis* in primary cultures of canine monocytes.

The above *in-vitro* culture technique made it possible for the production of sufficient quantities of whole cell antigen necessary for the development of the IFA procedure [31]. In view of the difficulty in detecting *E. canis* in the peripheral blood monocytes of infected dogs, the IFA test is the only method for the presumptive diagnosis of canine ehrlichiosis.

In-Vitro Cultivation and Studies of Ehrlichia sennetsu

Ehrlichia sennetsu was first cultivated *in vitro* by Sugi [1960] by using HeLa cells. Later, Minamishima [21] performed *in-vitro* studies on *E. sennetsu* with human amniotic membrane-derived FL cells, routinely grown in Melnick's medium. After successful cultivation of the microorganism for a lengthy period of time, it was concluded that the ehrlichia could replicate without interfering with host cell growth. There were possibly three factors that contributed to the maintenance of the FL cell culture in a persistently infected state [21]. First, the ehrlichial infection was not cytocidal. Secondly, the infected cells maintained the ability to divide, thereby facilitating cell-to-cell infection. Finally, there was a dense population of infected cells at each transfer. The persistence of the ehrlichia was confirmed by microscopic examination and titration in mice at each transfer. The virulence of the cultured ehrlichia was decreased as evidenced by an increase in the mean time to death of inoculated mice. Furthermore, the mean time to death of mice was substantially prolonged as the number of culture subpassages increased. These observations imply attenuation of the microorganism as a result of the continuous *in-vitro* cultivation in FL cells.

The Bs-C-1 line of *Cercopithecus* monkey kidney cells was also used for the *in-vitro* propagation of *E. sennstsu* [1]. The objective of the latter study was to compare various members of the rickettsia family to chlamydia and mycoplasma using the same cell culture. Unlike other rickettsiae, *E. sennetsu* were not found free in the cytoplasm but were contained in a vacuole within the host cell [1, 21]. Upon examination, the microorganisms were found to be extremely pleomorphic, having an average diameter ranging from 0.5 µm to 1.0 µm with some microorganisms being several micrometers in diameter [1] (Fig. 4). Morphological variations ranged from round to rod-shaped to various irregularly shaped bodies. Some infected cells contained a single microorganism or a pair of rod-shaped bacteria lying end-to-end, while others were heavily laden with various morphological forms. From this study, it was concluded

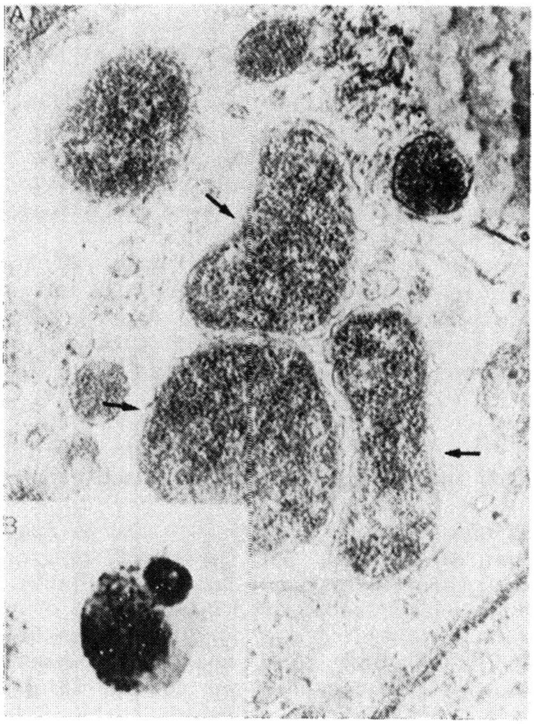

Figure 4. A. Electron micrograph of *Ehrlichia sennetsu* in P388D$_1$ cell cultures demonstrating the high degree of pleomorphism observed with this microorganism (arrows). B. Intracytoplasmic inclusions of *E. sennetsu* as observed in primary human monocyte cell cultures. Giemsa stain.

that there is little morphological evidence to support the initial hypothesis that *E. sennetsu* was related to the chlamydiae.

Electron microscopic examination of infected cells revealed that the ultrastructure of *E. sennetsu* may be similar to those of *R. prowazekii*, *R. rickettsii*, and *R. tsutsugamushi*. Each microorganism was bound by a rippled, tri-layered structure (the outer cell membrane) and a tri-layered plasma membrane. The internal structure showed evidence of prominent ribosomes and irregular patches that contained strands of DNA. The ground substance in some of the microorganisms was electron-dense and similar to the elementary bodies of the psittacosis agent, except for the lack of eccentric condensation of dense homogeneous material commonly observed in the latter [27]. Antigen yields from the above culture systems were insufficient, in comparison with other rickettsiae, for obtaining needed quantities of complement-fixing antigens and antigens for use in other more comprehensive studies [36].

Previous studies demonstrated that cyclophosphamide treatment of mice prior to infection enhances the growth of *E. sennetsu* [36]. Accordingly, Tachibana and his co-workers resorted to this method to procure soluble and particulate antigens of the agent [36]. Preliminary studies indicated that the primary constituent of the soluble antigens may be protein while the particulate antigen was, apparently, a non-protein substance. The soluble antigen was heat labile, whereas the particulate antigen was heat stable. In contrast, the soluble antigens of *R. prowazekii* and *R. rickettsii* are heat stable and their particulate antigens are heat labile [19]. Although the physiochemical properties of *E. sennetsu* are identical to those of *R. orientalis (Rickettsia tsutsugamushi)*, there was no cross-reaction in complement fixation tests [36].

Ehrlichia sennetsu was propagated successfully in primary human blood monocyte cultures [8] and primary canine blood monocyte cultures (Fig. 4A) [9, 11] by the technique developed by Nyindo et al., [23] for the propagation of *E. canis*. Both culture systems proved highly suitable for the *in-vitro* propagation of *E. sennetsu*. The microorganisms cultivated in canine monocyte cultures were used to develop an IFA test for seroepidemiology studies on sennetsu rickettsiosis [11]. Using this test system, some 3,000 human serum samples originating from Malaysia and other regions of Southeast Asia have been examined for the presence of anti-*E. sennetsu* antibodies. Approximately one-third of these sera, the majority of which were collected from patients with a febrile illness of undetermined etiology, contained *E. sennetsu*-specific

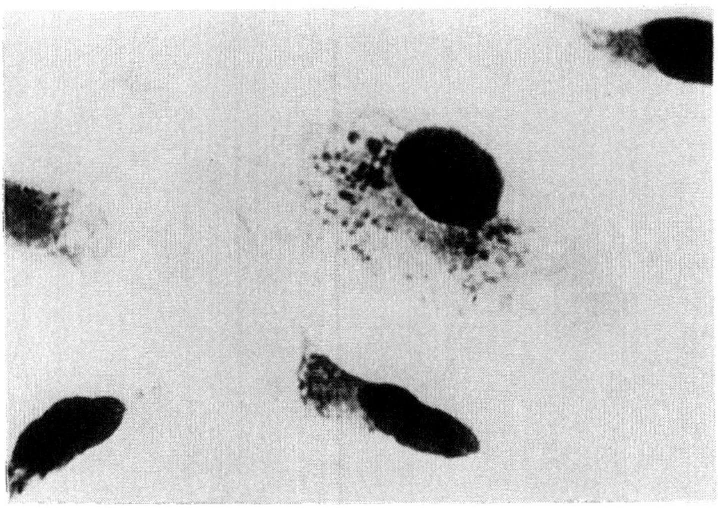

Figure 5. An *Ehrlichia sennetsu*-like agent isolated in P388D$_1$ cell cultures from the blood of a patient in Malaysia with fever of unknown origin. Serum from this patient reacted strongly in the IFA test with *E. sennetsu* antigen. Giemsa stain.

antibodies [11; Cole et al., unpublished results]. Three *E. sennetsu*-like agents have been isolated from whole blood samples collected from some of the above patients during the acute febrile stage of their illness (Fig. 5) [11]. Therefore, *E. sennetsu* or a antigenically related microorganism, present in Malaysia and possibly other regions of Southeast Asia, may be the cause of febrile illness. Due to the similarities of the clinical syndromes associated with infectious mononucleosis and sennetsu rickettsiosis, the latter disease may be present in other regions of the world, but remains undetected.

Ehrlichia sennetsu derived from the above canine monocyte culture system were subsequently used to establish infection in the continuous murine macrophage cell line $P388D_1$ [2]. Propagation of *E. sennetsu* in $P388D_1$ cells provided quantities of antigen suitable for various immunological and biochemical studies. Whole cells derived from $P388D_1$ cell cultures [38] were used in metabolism studies which showed that *E. sennetsu* utilizes glutamate at a much lower rate than the rickettsiae, but utilizes glutamine instead. These researchers also determined that *E. sennetsu* differs from *Wolbachia persica* and Chlamydiae, respectively, in that *E. sennetsu* cannot utilize glucose or glucose-6-phosphate. These results represent the first metabolic studies on any member of the genus *Ehrlichia*.

In a recent study, *E. sennetsu* and *E. canis* were separated from host-cell components by density gradient centrifugation. The antigenic structure of the purified whole cells was analysed by Western blot [25]. At least three polypeptides were common to the two bacteria, thereby confirming the earlier finding of an antigenic relationship between *E. sennetsu* and *E. canis*, determined by IFA [32].

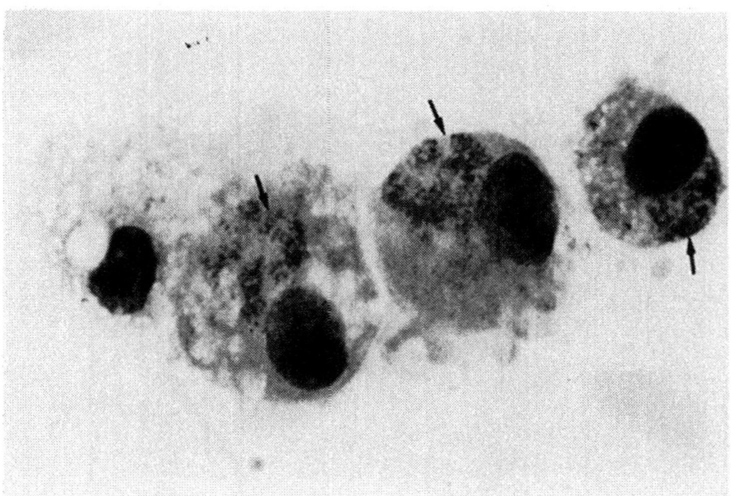

Figure 6. Inclusions of *Ehrlichia risticii* cultured in the $P388D_1$ cell line (arrows). Giemsa stain.

In-Vitro Cultivation of E. risticii

Ehrlichia risticii was initially isolated from the blood monocytes of a pony during the acute phase of PHF. The procedure employed isolation and cultivation techniques previously established for *E. canis* [23] and *E. sennetsu* [8, 11]. After the initial isolation in primary equine monocyte cultures, *E. risticii* was transferred and propagated in sequential primary canine blood monocyte cultures [10]. *Ehrlichia risticii* was then adapted successfully to continuous propagation in the murine macrophage cell line P388D_1 (Fig. 6) [12, 33], by techniques previously described for *E. sennetsu* [2]. The culture medium in this system consisted of medium 199 supplemented with 1% L-glutamine, 10% fetal bovine serum (FBS), and 5% sodium bicarbonate (5% w/v) (pH 7.2). Furthermore, the microorganisms have been propagated in the human histiocyte cell line, U937 [29]. Light and electron microscopy of *E. risticii*-infected cells revealed phenotypic characteristics typical of members of the genus *Ehrlichia* (Fig. 7) [12, 28].

Ehrlichia risticii-infected P388D_1 cells were used to develop an IFA test for seroepizootiologic studies and for the confirmatory serodiagnosis of PHF [33]. The large quantity of microorganisms generated by this culture system has facilitated various antigenic and physiologic studies [29, 38].

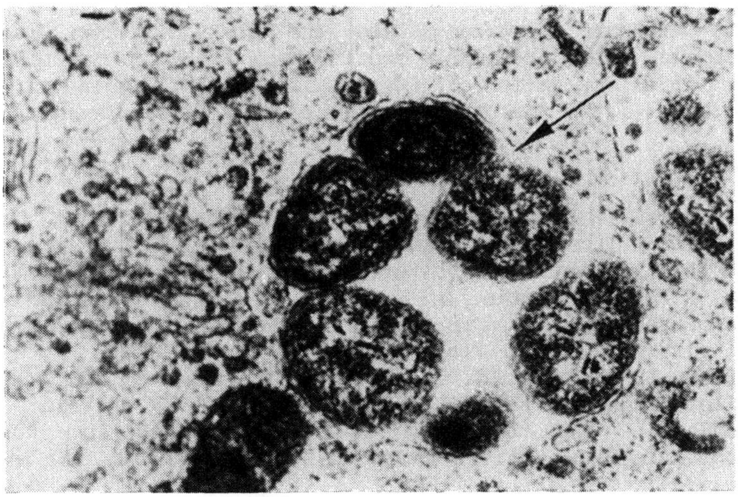

Figure 7. Electron micrograph of *Ehrlichia risticii* cultured in P388D_1 cells. The microorganisms contained within a cytoplasmic vacuole appear to replicate by binary fission (arrow).

Conclusion

Although *E. sennetsu*, previously believed to be a member of the genus *Rickettsia*, was the first ehrlichial agent to be cultured *in vitro* [35], it was 10 years before the genus *Ehrlichia* gained prominence. The etiology of TCP was clearly indicated prior to the development of the monocyte culture technique. However, the *in-vitro* cultivation of *E. canis* [23] further demonstrated the role of ehrlichiae in the etiology of a severe disease that devastated military working dogs during the Vietnam war. The biology and pathogenic potential of ehrlichiae were clearly recognized between 1970 and 1980. Various seroepizootiologic studies with culture-derived *E. canis* revealed that canine ehrlichiosis was a severe disease affecting dogs throughout the world [17,18]. Subsequently, a number of studies were carried out on various aspects of the disease, the microorganism and its mode of transmission, the antigenic structure, and effective chemotherapeutic measures [3, 5, 7, 16, 24, 25, 37]. Further antigenic structure studies on *E. canis* and *E. sennetsu* confirmed that the latter microorganism is a member of the genus *Ehrlichia*. Based upon knowledge gained in a relatively short period, a new ehrlichial pathogen was isolated from the blood of horses affected with the severe, often fatal, equine monocytic ehrlichiosis. The *in-vitro* propagation of *E. risticii* resulted in adequate quantities of microorganisms to conduct various immunologic studies, leading towards a better understanding of the antigenic structure of the genus *Ehrlichia*.

Recently, the host spectrum of the ehrlichiae has been extended to include humans [32]. Perhaps a modification of existing methods will lead to *in-vitro* propagation of the granulocytic ehrlichiae, *E. equi* and *E. phagocytophila*, and the purported human ehrlichiosis agent.

References

1. **Anderson, D., H. Hopps, M. Barile, and B. Berheim.** 1965. Comparison of the ultrastructure of several Rickettsia, Ornithosis virus and Mycoplasma in tissue culture. *J. Bacteriol.* **90**:1387-1404.
2. **Cole, A. I., M. Ristic, G. E. Lewis, Jr., and G. Rapmund.** 1985. Continuous propagation of *Ehrlichia sennetsu* in murine macrophage cell cultures. *Am. J. Trop. Med. Hyg.* **34**:774-780.
3. **Davidson, D. E., Jr., S. Dill Jr., M. Tingpalapong, S. Premaburtra, P. La-or Nguen, E. H. Stephenson, and M. Ristic.** 1978. Prophylactic and therapeutic use of tetracycline during an epizootic of ehrlichiosis among military dogs. *J. Am. Vet. Med. Assoc.* **172**:697-700.
4. **Donatien, A., and F. Lestoguard.** 1935. Existente en Algérie d'une Rickettsia du chien. *Bull. Soc. Pathol. Exot.* **28**:418-419.
5. **Groves, M., G. L. Dennis, H. L. Amyx, and D. L. Huxsoll.** 1975. Transmission of *Ehrlichia canis* to dogs by ticks (*Rhipicephalus sanguineus*). *Am. J. Vet. Res.* **36**:937-940.
6. **Hemelt, I. E., G. E. Lewis, Jr., D. L. Huxsoll, and E. H. Stephenson.** 1980. Serial propagation of *Ehrlichia canis* in primary canine peripheral blood monocyte cultures. *Cornell Vet.* **70**:37-42.

7. **Hildebrandt, P. K., J. D. Conroy, and A. E. McKee.** 1973. Ultrastructure of *Ehrlichia canis*. *Infect. Immun.* **7**:265-271.
8. **Hoilien, C. A., M. Ristic, D. L. Huxsoll, G. Rapmund, and N. Tachibana.** 1982. *Rickettsia sennetsu* in human blood monocyte cultures: similarities to the growth cycle of *Ehrlichia canis*. *Infect. Immun.* **35**:314-319.
9. **Holland, C. J.** 1980. *Rickettsia sennetsu* in canine monocyte cell cultures: development of a serodiagnostic test using culture-derived antigens. *M. S. Thesis.* University of Illinois, Urbana, IL.
10. **Holland, C. J., M. Ristic, A. I. Cole, P. Johnson, G. Baker, and T. Goetz.** 1985. Isolation, experimental transmission, and characterization of causative agent of Potomac horse fever. *Science* **227**:522-524.
11. **Holland, C. J., M. Ristic, D. L. Huxsoll, A. I. Cole, and G. Rapmund.** 1985a. Adaptation of *Ehrlichia sennetsu* to canine blood monocytes: Preliminary structural and serologic studies with cell culture-derived *Ehrlichia sennetsu*. *Infect. Immun.* **48**:366-371.
12. **Holland, C. J., E. Weiss, W. Burgdorfer, A. I. Cole, and I. Kakoma.** 1985b. *Ehrlichia risticii* sp. nov.: etiologic agent of equine monocytic ehrlichiosis (synonym, Potomac horse fever). *Int. J. Syst. Bacteriol.* **35**:524-526.
13. **Huxsoll, D. L., P. K. Hildebrandt, R. M. Nims, J. A. Ferguson, and J. S. Walker.** 1969. *Ehrlichia canis* - The causative agent of a haemorrhagic disease of dogs. *Vet. Rec.* **85**:587.
14. **Huxsoll, D. L., P. K. Hildebrandt, R. M. Nims, and J. S. Walker.** 1970a. Tropical canine pancytopenia. *J. Am. Vet. Med. Assoc.* **157**:1627-1632.
15. **Huxsoll, D. L., P. K. Hildebrandt, R. M. Nims, H. Amyx, and J. A. Ferguson.** 1970b. Epizootiology of tropical canine pancytopenia. *J. Wildl. Dis.* **6**:220-225.
16. **Kakoma, I., C. A. Carson, M. Ristic, D. L. Huxsoll, E. H. Stephenson, and M. B. A. Nyindo.** 1977. Autologous lymphocyte-mediated cytotoxicity against monocytes in canine ehrlichiosis. *Am. J. Vet. Res.* **38**:1557-1559.
17. **Keefe, T. J., C. J. Holland P. Salyer, and M. Ristic.** 1982. Distribution of *Ehrlichia canis* among military working dogs in the world and selected civilian dogs in the United States. *J. Am. Vet. Med. Assoc.* **181**:236-238.
18. **Knowles, R. C., D. W. Anderson, W. D. Shipley, R. H. Whitlock, B. D. Perry, and J. P. Davidson.** 1983. Acute equine diarrhea syndrome (AEDS): a preliminary report. *Proc. Am. Assoc. Equine Pract.* **29**:353-357.
19. **Kobayashi, Y.** 1969. Analytical serology of rickettsiae, pp. 203-256, *In* Analytical Serology of Microorganisms. J. B. G. Kwapinski, (Ed.) Vol. 1, John Wiley and Sons, Inc., NY.
20. **Lewis, G. E., Jr., D. L. Huxsoll, M. Ristic, and A. J. Johnson.** 1975. Experimentally induced infection of dogs, cats, and non-human primates with *Ehrlichia equi*, etiologic agent of equine ehrlichiosis. *Am. J. Vet. Res.* **36**:85-88.
21. **Minamishima, Y.** 1965. Persistent infection of *Rickettsia sennetsu* in cell culture system. *Jap. J. Microbiol.* **9**:75-86.

22. **Moulder, J. W.** 1974. The Rickettsias, pp. 882-928, *In* Bergey's Manual of Determinative Bacteriology. 8th edition. Williams and Wilkins, Baltimore, MD.
23. **Nyindo, M. B. A., M. Ristic, D. L. Huxsoll, and A. R. Smith.** 1971. Tropical canine pancytopenia: *in-vitro* cultivation of the causative agent - *Ehrlichia canis*. *Am. J. Vet. Res.* **32**:1651-1658.
24. **Nyindo, M. B. A., D. L. Huxsoll, M. Ristic, I. Kakoma, J. L. Brown, C. A. Carson, and E. H. Stephenson.** 1980. Cell mediated and humoral immune responses of German Shepherd dogs and beagles to experimental infection with *Ehrlichia canis*. *Am. J. Vet. Res.* **41**:250-254.
25. **Nyindo, M. B. A., I. Kakoma, C. J. Holland, R. Hansen, and M. Ristic.** 1989. Antigenic analysis of four *Ehrlichia spp.* by western immunoblot. *Am. J. Vet. Res.* In Press.
26. **Page, L. A.** 1974. Order II. Chlamydiales, pp. 914-918, *In* Bergey's Manual of Determinative Bacteriology, R. E. Buchanan and N. E. Gibbons (Eds.). 8th edition. Williams and Wilkens, Baltimore, MD.
27. **Rake, G.** 1957. Family II. Clamydiaceae, *In* Bergey's Manual of Determinative Bacteriology, Breed, Murry and Smith (Eds). 7th edition. Williams and Wilkins, Baltimore, MD.
28. **Rikihisa, Y., B. D. Perry, and D. D. Cordes.** 1985. Ultrastructural study of ehrlichial organisms in the large colons of ponies infected with Potomac horse fever. *Infect. Immun.* **49**:505-512.
29. **Rikihisa, Y., and B. M. Jiang.** 1988. *In vitro* susceptibility of *Ehrlichia risticii* to eight antibiotics. *Antimicrob. Agents Chemother.* **32**:986-991.
30. **Ristic, M., and D. L. Huxsoll.** 1984. *Ehrlichieae, In* Bergey's Manual of Systematic Bacteriology, N. R. Krieg (Ed.). Vol. 1. Williams and Wilkens, Baltimore, MD.
31. **Ristic, M., D. L. Huxsoll, R. M. Weisiger, P. K. Hildebrandt, and M. B. A. Nyindo.** 1972. Serological diagnosis of tropical canine pancytopenia by indirect immunofluorescence. *Infect. Immun.* **6**:226-231.
32. **Ristic, M., D. L. Huxsoll, N. Tachibana, and G. Rapmund.** 1981. Evidence of a serologic relationship between *Ehrlichia canis* and *Rickettsia sennetsu*. *Am. J. Trop. Med. Hyg.* **30**:1324-1328.
33. **Ristic, M., C. J. Holland, J. E. Dawson, J. Sessions, and J. E. Palmer.** 1986. Diagnosis of equine monocytic ehrlichiosis (syn. Potomac horse fever) by indirect immunofluorescence. *Am. J. Vet. Res.* **49**:1497-1500.
34. **Smith, R. D., and M. Ristic.** 1977. Ehrlichia, pp.295-328, *In* Parasitic protozoa IV. J. P. Kreier (Ed.). Academic Press, Inc., NY.
35. **Sugi, Y.** 1960. Tissue culture of the pathogenic agent of glandular fever. *Fukuoka Acta Med.* **51**:1056-1060.
36. **Tachibana, N., T. Kusaba, I. Matsumoto, and Y. Kobayashi.** 1975. Purification of complement-fixing antigens of *Rickettsia sennetsu* by ether treatments. *Infect. Immun.* **13**:1030-1036.

37. **Weisiger, R. M., M. Ristic, and D. L. Huxsoll.** 1975. Kinetics of antibody response to *Ehrlichia canis* assayed by the indirect fluorescent antibody method. *Am. J. Vet. Res.* **36**:689-694.
38. **Weiss, E., G. A. Dasch, Y. H. Kang, and H. N. Westfall.** 1988. Substrate utilization by *Ehrlichia sennetsu* and *Ehrlichia risticii* separated from host constituents by Renografin gradient centrifugation. *J. Bacteriol.* **170**:5012-5017.

3. ULTRASTRUCTURE OF RICKETTSIAE WITH SPECIAL EMPHASIS ON EHRLICHIAE

YASUKO RIKIHISA, Ph.D.

Abstract

Basic morphological features of rickettsiae and ehrlichiae are similar to those of gram-negative bacteria. The uptake and intracellular fates of the rickettsiae in eukaryotic cells are markedly different. For example, *Rickettsia tsutsugamushi* cells are individually phagocytized by polymorphonuclear leukocytes in tightly enclosed phagosomal membranes. Lysosomes, labeled with electron-dense tracers or by acid phosphatase cytochemistry, do not fuse with the bacteria-laden phagosomes. Subsequently, the microorganisms are released from phagosomes into the host cytoplasm. *Ehrlichia risticii*, the etiologic agent of Potomac horse fever, infects macrophages and glandular epithelial cells of the intestines of horses. The microorganisms are pleomorphic and exist as two distinct morphological forms. The small forms (0.2 to 0.4 µm in diameter) are electron-dense and some were undergoing binary fission. Multiple small forms of the microorganisms occur in loosely enclosed host membrane vacuoles. On the other hand, larger forms (0.6 to 1.5 µm in diameter) are less electron-dense and individual microorganisms are tightly enveloped by host membranes. In contrast, *Cowdria ruminantium*, which belongs to the tribe Ehrlichiae, was found in loosely enclosed host membrane vacuoles. Lysosomal fusion with bacteria-laden vacuoles was not detectable. Rickettsial antigens were demonstrated in the capsular layer by immunoferritin labeling. The capsular component appeared extremely abundant in *C. ruminantium*. The outer membrane of rickettsiae has a thick outer leaflet (*R. tsutsugamushi*) or inner leaflet (*R. prowazekii* and *R. rickettsii*). The outer membrane of ehrlichiae does not show this variation in thickness. Rickettsiae, ehrlichiae, and *C. ruminantium* produce outer membrane vesicles of variable sizes in the host cell. A peptidoglycan layer in the periplasmic space is not obvious in rickettsiae or ehrlichiae. However, *C. ruminantium* had a large amount of peptidoglycan-like material between the outer and inner membrane. Although the rickettsial and ehrlichial microorganisms show similarities in their basic morphology, they vary markedly in their capsule, outer membrane, and peptidoglycan structure.

Introduction

The ultrastructure of the bacteria of the genus *Rickettsia* varies depending upon the culture conditions, the host cell infected, whether the infection is carried out *in-vitro* or *in-vivo*, and the electron microscopic method of preparation of samples for analysis [3]. Additional variables that influence the ultrastructure of rickettsia include the strains, serovars, and biovars. In this presentation the

J. C. Williams and I. Kakoma (eds.), Ehrlichiosis, 22–31.

ultrastructural data on the genus *Ehrlichia* will be discussed in comparison with that of the genus *Rickettsia*.

Materials and Methods

Culture of Ehrlichiae. *Ehrlichia risticii* was cultured in a human monocyte-like histiocytic lymphoma cell line U-937 [13, 14] or murine macrophage cell line $P388D_1$ [21] as previously described [13, 14, 21]. Experiments for examining lysosomal fusion were performed as described previously [8, 10, 21].

Infection of Ponies with Ehrlichia risticii. Ponies were experimentally infected by the intravenous injection of 1 x 10^7 to 4 x 10^7 *E. risticii*-infected U-937 or $P388D_1$ cells. Rectal temperatures and clinical signs were recorded daily. The ponies were euthanized a few days after they developed diarrhea, and tissue specimens were immediately processed for electron microscopy [15].

Infection of Goats with Cowdria ruminantium. The animals were infected and housed in strict isolation rooms at the United States Drug Administration Plum Island facility. Goats were injected intravenously with 4 ml of blood collected from a febrile goat that was experimentally infected with the *C. ruminantium* Mali 1 strain [4] or mouse-adapted Kumm strain (kindly provided by J. L. DuPlessis). Rectal temperatures were recorded daily. The goats were observed closely and, in the event of death, a postmortem was immediately performed. The cranium was opened and the brain was removed. Small tissue specimens from the choroid plexus were dissected and minced in fixative. Horse and goat tissue specimens and cultured infected cells were processed for transmission electron microscopy as previously described [3]. In all cases, every effort was made to save the animals according to recommendations for humane use of experimental animals.

Results and Discussion

Ehrlichia risticii

Ehrlichia risticii is the primary etiologic bacterium of Potomac horse fever. The bacterium is found in the cells of the mucosa and submucosa of the colon, cecum, and, to a lesser extent, small intestine of infected horses [6, 15, 21]. Although the microorganism could be isolated in tissue culture from blood monocytes and the spleen of infected horses [13, 14], it was difficult to identify the bacteria by transmission electron microscopy. In the equine intestine, macrophages, glandular epithelial cells, and mast cells were infected [6, 15, 16]. Microorganisms occurred as clusters in the cytoplasmic phagosomes of macrophages [20] or in the apical cytoplasm in phagosomes of crypt epithelial cells, including mitotic cells near the bottom of the gland. In mast cells, *E. risticii* were difficult to see by light microscopy due to the presence of overwhelming numbers of mast cell granules. Under the light microscope, each cluster of *E. risticii* appeared to be contained within a single phagosomal vacuole. In most cases, however, microorganisms were individually enveloped in separate phagosomal vacuoles.

Ehrlichia risticii cells were highly pleomorphic and heterogeneous in electron density [6, 15, 16]. Although the majority of *E. risticii* were round, bizarre-shaped microorganisms were present, especially during *in-vitro* cultivation. Most *E. risticii* in intestinal glandular epithelial cells and macrophages were electron-lucent large bacteria (0.6-1.5 µm in diameter) individually wrapped in host vacuolar membranes [6, 15, 16]. There was very little space between the host vacuolar membrane and the outer membrane of these electron-lucent microorganisms [6, 15, 16], (Fig. 1), making it difficult to identify the host vacuolar membrane at

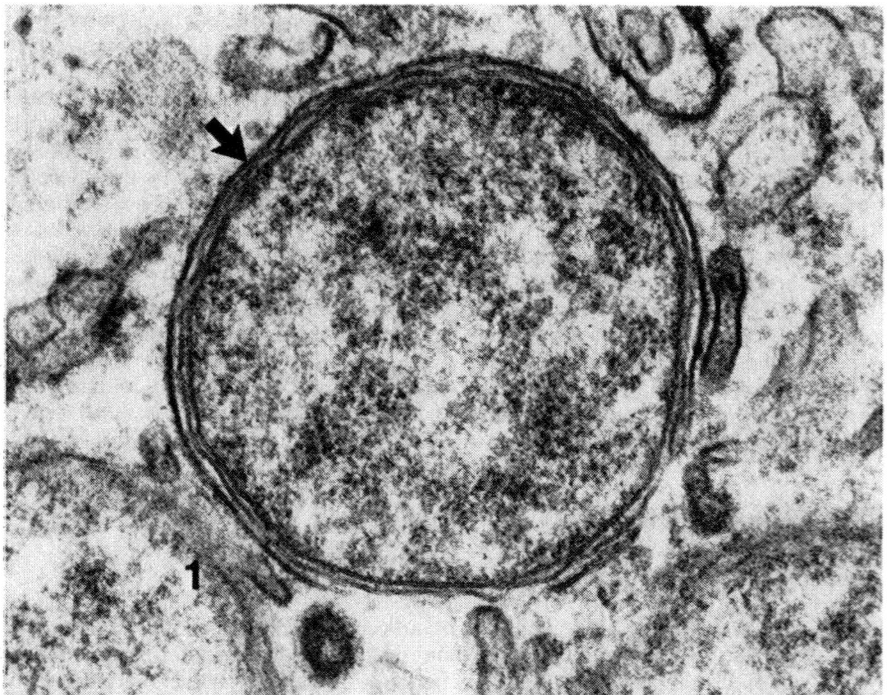

Figure 1. Appearance of *Ehrlichia risticii* in equine intestinal glandular epithelial cells or macrophages. A large electron-lucent form of *E. risticii* tightly wrapped in host vacuolar membrane. Note the similar thickness of three membranes: host vacuolar (arrow), and outer and inner membranes of *E. risticii*. There is no thickening of the inner and outer leaflets of the outer membrane. Ribosomes and DNA filaments are clearly seen. X 105,000.

low magnification. A similar association between phagosomal membranes and the outer membrane of *R. tsutsugamushi* was reported previously [7, 10]. Electron-dense smaller bacteria (0.2-0.4 μm in diameter) were seen less frequently in infected equine intestine than in U-937 [13, 14] or $P388D_1$ macrophages [21]. The electron density of the smaller bacteria was partially due to more tightly packed ribosomes. Under the electron microscope, electron-dense bacteria were much easier to detect, because their contrast against host tissue background was higher than that of electron-lucent microorganisms. A vacuolar membrane loosely surrounded morulae with multiple electron-dense bacteria in the same vacuole, including those microorganisms in the process of transverse binary fission [13, 14, 21]. Phagosomal vacuoles were usually small, containing 5-20 microorganisms per vacuole in ultrathin section. Gigantic phagolysosomal vacuoles containing 50 or more microorganisms, as are seen with *Coxiella burnetii* [1], were not observed with *E. risticii*. When electron-dense and electron-lucent bacteria occurred within the same vacuole, the electron-lucent microorganisms were always located peripherally and were tightly attached to the vacuolar membrane [15] (Fig. 2), thus, suggesting that electron-lucent bacteria had an

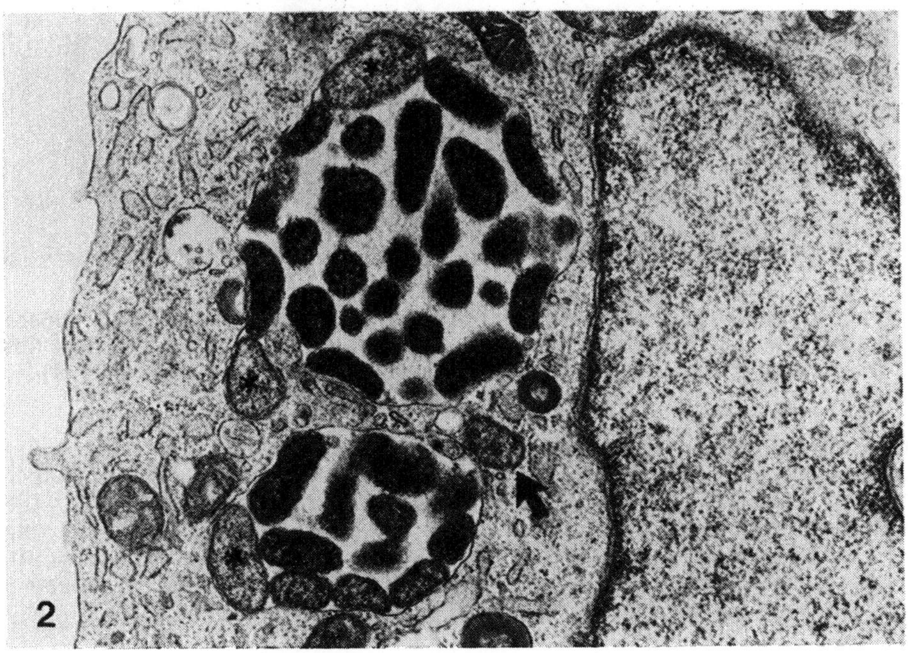

Figure 2. *Ehrlichia risticii* propagated in U-937 cell culture. Two vacuoles containing both electron-lucent (*) and electron-dense forms. The electron-lucent forms (*) are always located peripherally in the vacuole. Some are tightly wrapped in host membrane (arrow). X 24,000.

affinity for the host membrane. Occasionally observed were multiple microorganisms that were tightly enveloped within a continuous host membrane of which the sites of continuity were short, narrow stalks (Fig. 3). These figures suggest that the electron-dense smaller bacterium increases its surface area by swelling within the vacuole.

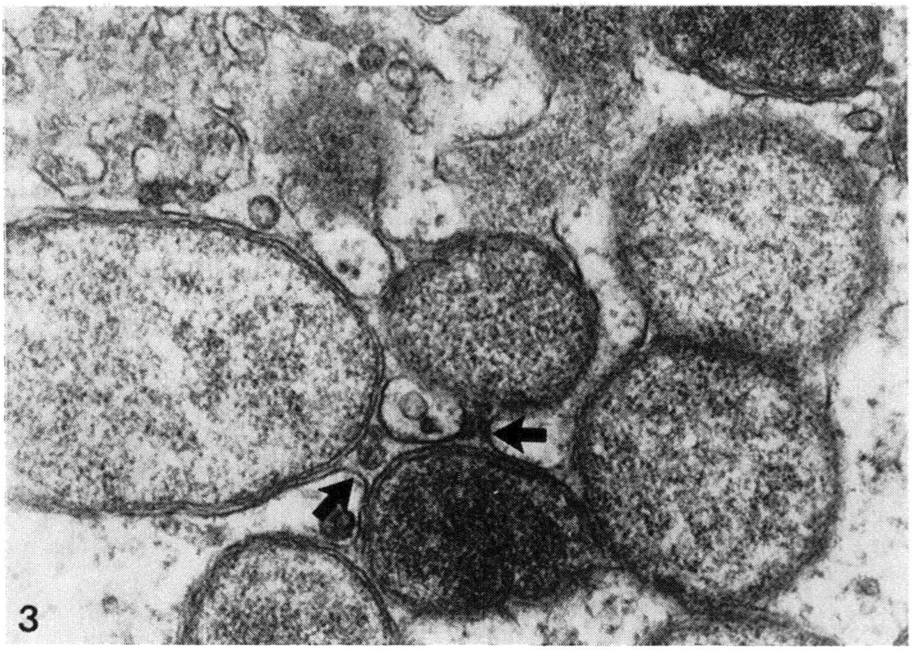

Figure 3. Multiple *Ehrlichia risticii*, which vary in their ribosomal content, are enveloped by continuous host membrane. The site of host-membrane continuity appears to form short narrow stalks (arrows). X 56,000.

These changes were accompanied by a concomitant development of a close association with the vacuolar membrane and a subsequent pinching-off of tightly invested vacuoles. Recondensation of electron-lucent large cells into electron-dense small cells, as seen in chlamydiae [5], were not observed with *E. risticii*. Electron-dense microorganisms in a single vacuole were seldom seen. Such electron-dense bacteria were not seen among *R. tsutsugamushi*-infected eukaryotic cells [3, 7, 8, 9, 10, 11, 18].

The fate of ehrlichia-laden phagosomes was followed by the cytochemical detection of acid phosphatase and by examination of the fusion with tracer-preloaded phagolysosomes [21]. Ehrlichia-laden phagosomes did not fuse with lysosomes in $P388D_1$ cells [21]. However, rapid abrogation of inhibition of lysosomal fusion took place when 10 μg/ml oxytetracycline was added to *E. risticii*-infected P388D_1 cells [21]. When *R. tsutsugamushi* was phagocytized by polymorphonuclear leukocytes (PMN), lysosomal fusion with phagosomes containing intact bacteria was not evident. These intact bacteria subsequently escaped from the phagosomes to the cytoplasm of the PMN [7, 8, 10]. Lysosomal fusion was evident, however, when bacteria were inactivated at 56°C for 30 min. These inactivated bacteria were eventually disintegrated. Viable chlamydiae were also reported to inhibit lysosomal fusion [5].

Outer and inner membranes of *E. risticii* were similar in thickness. The outer membrane did not show thickening of inner or outer leaflets and a peptidoglycan layer was not evident. A lipopolysaccharide or capsular layer, however, was evident on the surface of electron-dense bacteria [14, 15], but was not evident in electron-lucent microorganisms, as the phagosomal and outer membranes were too closely associated to permit such an observation. Members of the genus *Rickettsia* showed thickening of the outer (*R. tsutsugamushi*) or inner (*R. rickettsii, R. prowazekii*) leaflet [19]. *Coxiella burnetii* showed thickening of the inner leaflet of the outer membrane [2]. Surface antigen was detectable by immunoferritin labeling [18] of *R. tsutsugamushi* and *E. risticii* [17]. Outer membrane vesicles were seen

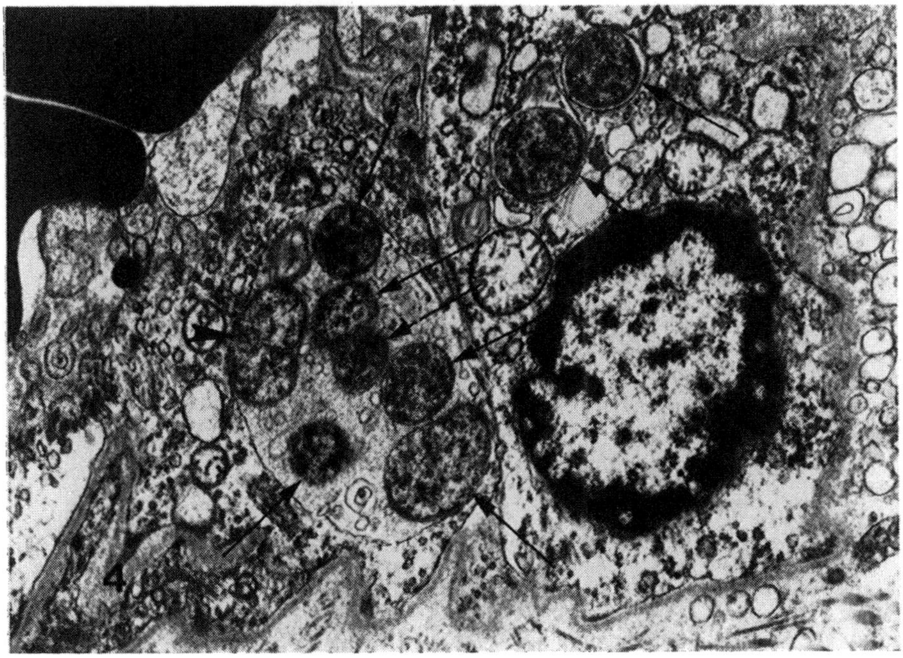

Figure 4. A. Electron micrograph of *Ehrlichia sennetsu* in P388D_1 cell cultures demonstrating the high degree of pleomorphism observed with this microorganism (arrows). B. Intracytoplasmic inclusions of *E. sennetsu* as observed in primary human monocyte cell cultures. Giemsa stain.

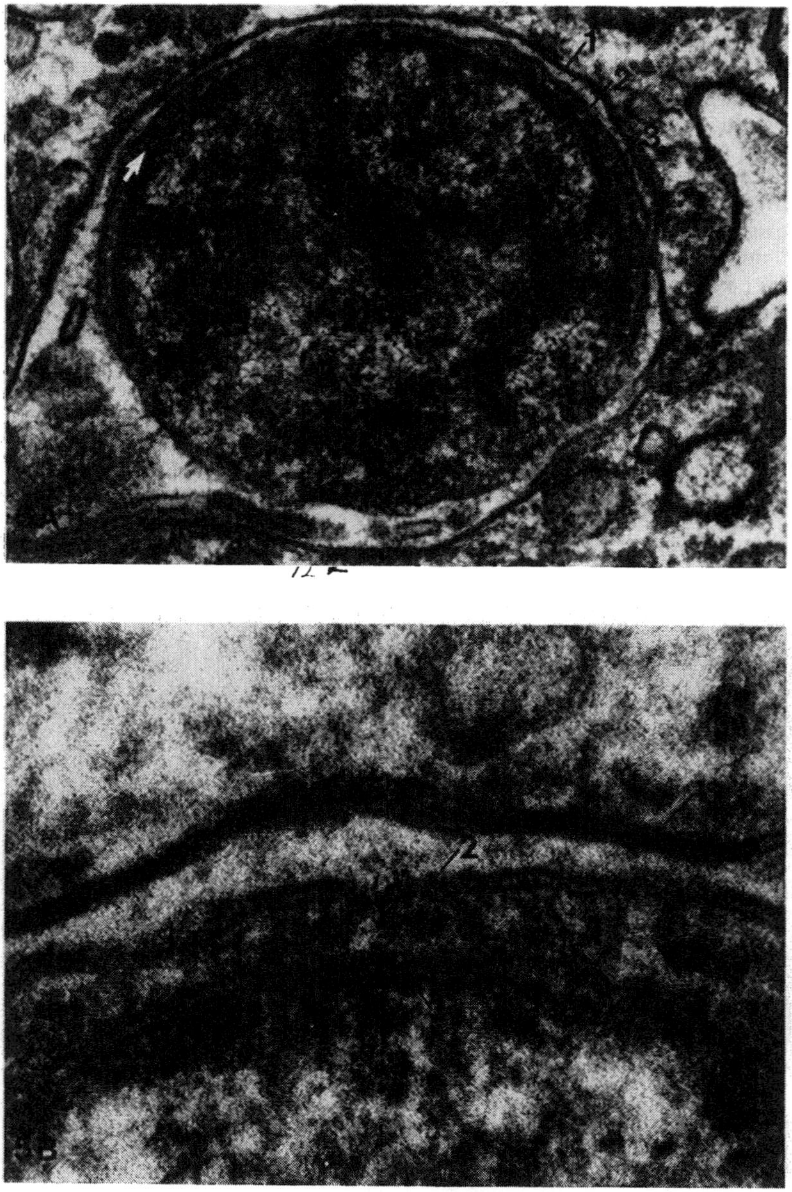

Figure 5. Ultrastructure of *Cowdria ruminantium* grown in goat endothelial cells. High magnification of *C. ruminantium* Mali 1 strain. The microorganism is surrounded by two layers of unit membrane. Inner (3) and outer (2) membranes are almost the same thickness as the host vacuolar membrane (1). In the periplasmic space, electron-dense substance is evident (arrow). A X 102,000, B X 500,000.

with *R. tsutsugamushi* [9]. Similar membrane vesicles and smaller membrane vesicles containing electron-dense substance were occasionally seen with *E. risticii* in the host vacuoles [15]. These vesicles were more frequently seen in degenerating host cells.

Cowdria ruminantium

In the choroid plexus of goats experimentally infected with Mali 1 [4] or Kumm strain of *C. ruminantium*, both strains were found in the phagosomal vacuoles of endothelial cells [12]. Multiple cowdriae tended to occur in large vacuoles, although occasionally single microorganisms were seen in small vacuoles [12], (Fig. 4). The size of the vacuole and the number of microorganisms per vacuole were generally larger than those observed with ehrlichiae. The cowdriae were round and there was more space between the vacuolar membrane and the microorganisms than with the ehrlichiae [12], (Fig. 4). The abundant capsular components appeared as an amorphous gray substance in the cowdriae-laden vacuole (Fig. 4), [4]. Two bacterial forms, electro-dense and -lucent, were not evident in cowdriae. A peptidoglycan-like material was extremely abundant in the periplasmic spaces of both Kumm and Mali 1 strains [12] (Fig. 5). In some sections, the amount of periplasmic space was larger than the cytoplasm of the bacteria [12]. The inner membrane was smooth, but the outer membrane was wavy, and outpouchings were present at single or multiple sites due to the presence of a large quantity of peptidoglycan-like material in the periplasm (Fig. 6). Thickening of

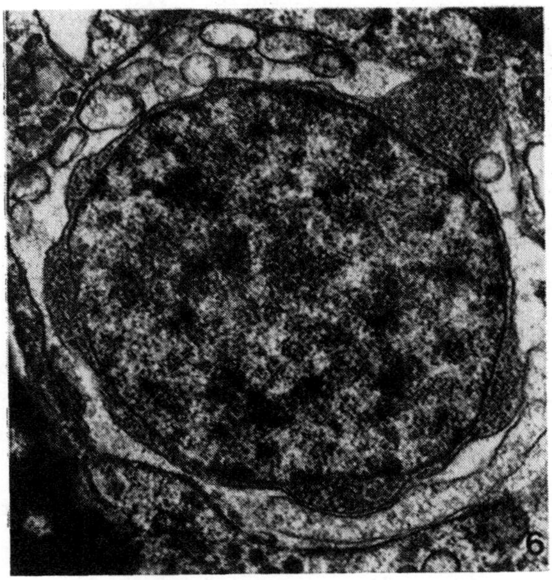

Figure 6. *Cowdria ruminantium* Mali 1 strain grown in the cytoplasmic vacuole of caprine endothelial cells. Note the undulating outer membrane and periplasm packed with peptidoglycan-like material. X 48,000.

either leaflet of the outer membrane was absent [12], (Fig. 5). Although cowdriae and ehrlichiae belong to the tribe *Ehrlichieae*, their ultrastructures are significantly different.

Acknowledgements

The work with *C. ruminantium* was carried out in collaboration with Dr. Linda L. Logan. A portion of this work was supported by USDA grant 85-CRJR-2-2593.

References

1. **Baca, O. G., and D. Paretsky.** 1983. Q fever and *Coxiella burnetii*: a model for host-parasite interactions. *Microbiol. Rev.* **47**:127-149.
2. **Burton, P. R., J. Stueckemann, and D. Paretsky.** 1975. Electron microscopy studies of the limiting layers of the rickettsia *Coxiella burnetii*. *J. Bacteriol.* **122**:316-324.
3. **Ito, S., and Y. Rikihisa.** 1981. Techniques for electron microscopy of rickettsiae, *In* W. Burgdorfer and R. L. Anacker (eds.), *Rickettsiae and Rickettsial Diseases*, Academic Press, pp. 213-227.
4. **Logan, L. L., Y. Rikihisa, T. J. Galvin, and M. Toure.** 1989. The isolation of *Cowdria ruminantium* from *Amblyomma variegatum* collected in Mali. (In preparation).
5. **Moulder, J. W.** 1984. Looking at chlamydiae without looking at their hosts. *Am. Soc. Microbiol. News.* **50**:353-362.
6. **Rikihisa, Y.** 1986. Ultrastructural studies of ehrlichial organisms in the organs of ponies with equine monocytic ehrlichiosis (synonym, Potomac Horse Fever), *In* H. Winkler and M. Ristic (eds). *Microbiology 1986,* American Society for Microbiology, Washington, DC, pp. 200-202.
7. **Rikihisa, Y., and S. Ito.** 1979. Intracellular localization of *R. tsutsugamushi* in polymorphonuclear leukocytes. *J. Exp. Med.* **150**:703-708.
8. **Rikihisa, Y., and S. Ito.** 1980. Localization of electron dense tracers during entry of *Rickettsia tsutsugamushi* into polymorphonuclear leukocytes. *Infect. Immun.* **30**:231-242.
9. **Rikihisa, Y., and S. Ito.** 1981. Outer membrane vesicles of *Rickettsia tsutsugamushi* in baby hamster kidney cells. *In* W. Burgdorfer and R. L. Anacker (eds.), *Rickettsiae and Rickettsial Diseases*, Academic Press, pp. 229-240.
10. **Rikihisa, Y., and S. Ito.** 1982. Mechanism of entry of *Rickettsia tsutsugamushi* into polymorphonuclear leukocytes. *Infect. Immun.* **38**:343-350.
11. **Rikihisa, Y., and S. Ito.** 1983. Effect of antibody on entry of *Rickettsia tsutsugamushi* into polymorphonuclear leukocytes. *Infect. Immun.* **39**:928-938.
12. **Rikihisa, Y., and L. L. Logan.** 1986. Unusual peptidoglycan substance in *Cowdria ruminantium* in the endothelial cells of the

choroid plexus of the goat. *Proc. XIth Int. Cong. on Electron Microscopy*, pp. 3345-3346.

13. **Rikihisa, Y., and B. D. Perry.** 1984. Causative agent of Potomac horse fever. *Vet. Rec.* **115**:554.
14. **Rikihisa, Y., and B. D. Perry.** 1985. Causative ehrlichial organisms in Potomac horse fever. *Infect. Immun.* **49**:513-517.
15. **Rikihisa, Y., B. D. Perry, and D. O. Cordes.** 1985. Ultrastructural study of rickettsial organisms in the large colon of ponies experimentally infected with Potomac horse fever. *Infect. Immun.* **49**:505-512.
16. **Rikihisa, Y., B. D. Perry, and D. O. Cordes.** 1984. Rickettsial link with acute equine diarrhea. *Vet. Rec.* **115**:390.
17. **Rikihisa, Y., C. I. Pretzman, G. C. Johnson, S. M. Reed, S. Yamamoto, and F. Andrews.** 1988. Clinical, pathologic and immunological responses of ponies to *Ehrlichia sennetsu* and subsequent *Ehrlichia risticii* challenge. *Infect. Immun.* **56**:2960-2966.
18. **Rikihisa, Y., T. R. Rota, A. B. MacDonald, and S. Ito.** 1979. Changes in immunoferritin labeling of *Rickettsia tsutsugamushi* after serial cultivation in ^{60}Co-irradiated BHK-21 cells. *Infect. Immun.* **26**:638-650.
19. **Silverman, D. J., and C. L. Wisseman, Jr.** 1978. Comparative ultrastructural study on the cell envelopes of *Rickettsia prowazekii, Rickettsia rickettsii*, and *Rickettsia tsutsugamushi*. *Infect. Immun.* **21**:1020-1023.
20. **Steele, K., Y. Rikihisa, and A. Walton.** 1986. Demonstration of *Ehrlichia* in Potomac horse fever using a silver stain. *Vet. Pathol.* **23**:531-533.
21. **Wells, M. Y., and Y. Rikihisa.** 1988. Lack of lysosomal fusion with phagosomes containing *Ehrlichia risticii* in $P388D_1$ cells: Abrogation of inhibition with oxytetracycline. *Infect. Immun.* **56**:3209-3215.

4. ANTIGENIC PROPERTIES OF THE EHRLICHIAE AND OTHER RICKETTSIACEAE

G. A. DASCH, Ph.D.
E. WEISS, Ph.D.
J. C. Williams, Ph.D.

Abstract

The family Rickettsiaceae consists of a diverse group of small gram-negative bacteria, most of which show intimate association with diverse arthropods and exhibit obligate intracellular growth. The chemical and antigenic properties of members of the tribe Rickettsieae (*Rickettsia, Rochalimaea, Coxiella*) are understood relatively well in contrast to those of the tribe Ehrlichieae (*Ehrlichia, Cowdria, Neorickettsia*) or the poorly known tribe Wolbachieae (*Wolbachia, Rickettsiella*). With the advent of improved *in-vitro* cultivation systems for an increasing number of Rickettsiaceae, quality preparations of these diverse bacteria can now be obtained routinely by procedures such as Renografin or Percoll density gradient centrifugation. The availability of purified preparations has permitted the initiation of studies of the molecular and antigenic properties of the unique genus- and species-specific antigens. We present a brief review of the Rickettsiaceae with regard to current progress achieved in the chemical characterization of purified lipopolysaccharide and protein antigens, Western blotting comparisons of antigens with both polyclonal and monoclonal antibodies, and the molecular cloning and sequencing of DNA encoding different protein antigens. The phylogenetic implications for the Rickettsiaceae of the determination of the sequences of the conserved 60-kDa heat-shock proteins (Hsp 60) and 16S ribosomal RNAs are also considered.

Diversity Of Microorganisms Placed In The Rickettsiaceae

The last taxonomic treatment of the Order Rickettsiales appeared 5 years ago [95]. At that time it was acknowledged that the order was exceedingly complex (Fig. 1) and that the data base available for most of the bacteria placed in the order was inadequate for a rational classification. It is striking that the percentage of characteristics used in the taxonomy of Rickettsiales, which are based on the nature of host-cell associations (cellular location, cell type, vertebrate or invertebrate growth), or on medical or veterinary considerations (pathogenicity, arthropod host, geography), far outnumbered specific characterisitics of the bacteria as microorganisms.

At present, these statements are still true with regard to the subdivision of the Order Rickettsiales into the families Bartonellaceae, Anaplasmataceae, and Rickettsiaceae and their classification (Fig. 1). The family Anaplasmataceae includes four genera and 13 species of obligately parasitic bacteria which lack trilaminar cell walls and which

J. C. Williams and I. Kakoma (eds.), Ehrlichiosis, 32–58.

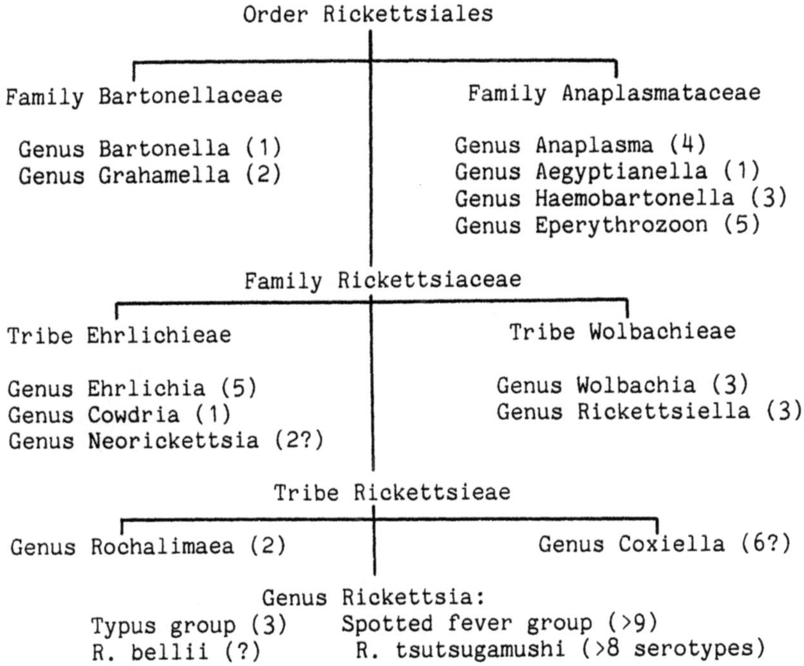

Figure 1. Schematic of current taxonomic arrangement of the Order Rickettsiales. The present number of described species or major genotypic variants (?) that may be distinct species is indicated in parentheses after each genus.

grow in intimate association with vertebrate erythrocytes. The small family Bartonellaceae contains two genera and three species which are cultivable, contain trilaminar cell walls, and although erythrocyte-associated like the Anaplasmataceae, appear to have a broader range of cell associations than the latter. No molecular studies relating these two families have been reported.

On the other hand, some trends are becoming clear among the large number of species in the largest family in the Order Rickettsiales, the Rickettsiaceae. It is currently divided into three tribes, eight genera and at least 27 species (Fig. 1). The advent of improved methods for the cultivation, purification, and molecular characterization of minute quantities of antigens and DNA from representative species of Rickettsiaceae have led to a revolution in our microbiological understanding of these species. In particular, the properties of the conserved 16S ribosomal RNA and 60-kDa heat-shock proteins (Hsp 60) of the Rickettsiaceae have clearly demonstrated the polyphyletic associations of these species. The full ramifications of these studies, both for the taxonomic status of the Rickettsiaceae and for our fundamental understanding of the microbiological properties and evolutionary history of each species, are just now being perceived.

Improved Methodology For Characterizing Rickettsiaceae

The improved microbiological understanding of Rickettsiaceae in the past 5 years can be attributed directly to improved methods of cultivation, purification, and characterizaton of these bacteria. Although both continuous cell culture and yolk sac culture methods have been long employed with the Rickettsieae and *Wolbachia persica* [90], the adaptation of *Ehrlichia sennetsu* and *E. risticiii* to continuous culture in mouse $P388D_1$ cells [14] has permitted the routine production of significant amounts of these bacteria for the first time. Ehrlichiae, *N. helminthoeca*, and *Cowdria ruminantium* have been grown in primary tissue culture systems [30, 45, 52, 105]. *Rickettsiella* has been grown for limited periods in continuous mammalian cell culture [75]. The lack of extensive microbiological characterization of these species as well as other species of *Wolbachia, Ehrlichia*, and *Rickettsiella* is attributable in large part to the lack of highly productive continuous tissue culture sytems for their routine growth. Some progress has been made in this area. Recently, propagation of three of four isolates of *Cowdria ruminantium* was achieved in a continuous calf endothelial cell system, which may permit mass propagation of this agent [8]. Recently, Woldehiwet and Scott [107] succeeded in cultivating *Cytoecetes phagocytophila,* the etiologic agent of tick-borne fever. Both human fibroblast-dog macrophage and mouse-dog hybrid cell lines have been described for propagating *E. canis* [64, 72]. Once such culture systems have been improved and are more widely available, the application of the methodological improvements achieved with other Rickettsiaceae should permit their rapid microbiological characterization.

The separation of Rickettsiaceae from host cell components by ultracentrifugation in either Renografin or Percoll density gradients has been instrumental for the routine investigation of the physiology, biochemistry, and immunology of these species. Although *R. typhi, R. prowazekii*, and *Coxiella burnetii* can be obtained essentially free of host cell components [23, 91, 99] with the Renografin technique, spotted fever group rickettsiae retain small amounts of host cell contaminants (104, Dasch, unpublished observations). Moreover, both the monocytic ehrlichiae and scrub typhus rickettsiae have resisted complete purification with either Percoll or Renografin techniques [20, 24, 77, 92, 93, 96]. These fundamental differences in cell-association properties of these bacteria are poorly understood and have necessitated the use of extensive controls for interpreting the experimental results obtained with such partially purified materials [92, 93, 96]. Three additional methods have been developed that have particular utility for antigenic and recombinant DNA approaches to the characterization of *Rickettsia* and *Ehrlichia*. Repeated freeze/thaw treatment of heavily infected tissue culture suspensions followed by Sephacryl S-1000 column chromatography has provided nonviable preparations suitable for use in enzyme-linked immunosorbent assay (ELISA) or for preparation of DNA for genomic cloning and restriction fragment length polymorphism (RFLP) analysis [56, 57]. A simple Triton X-100 release method for preparing rickettsial DNA suitable for RFLP and polymerase chain reaction (PCR) analysis has also been developed [61, 62]. A rapid micromethod for purifying viable extracellular *R. typhi* and spotted fever group rickettsiae has also been used to analyze the antigenic variation in these species by Western blotting [22, 58-60].

Classical chemical, biochemical, and immunological methods for analyzing isolated bacteria have been used to determine the microbiological properties of some Rickettsiaceae. The most information has been obtained about *Coxiella* and typhus-group rickettsiae, as they can be obtained in relatively large quantities and good purity. Antigenic analysis by radioimmunoprecipitation or Western blotting analysis with both monoclonal and polyclonal sera have also provided more comprehensive comparisons between strains, species, and genera. Finally, direct analysis of DNA by RFLP or PCR methods, or most powerfully, the cloning, replication, and sequencing of isolated genes or DNA fragments from genomic libraries created in lambda, cosmid, or plasmid vectors of *E. coli* have provided the deepest insights into the microbiology of the Rickettsiaceae.

Characteristics Of Lipopolysaccharide Among Rickettsiaceae

Lipopolysaccharide (LPS) is one of the major antigens present in the cell wall of gram-negative eubacteria and is responsible for a large amount of the serological variation found in these microorganisms (the somatic O-type heat-stable serotypes). With the major exception of *Rickettsia tsutsugamushi*, which lacks detectable LPS [2], LPS-like molecules have been readily demonstrable in all of the Rickettsiaceae that have been investigated with appropriate methods (Table 1). By

TABLE 1. Lipoploysaccharides of Rickettsiaceae.

Group or genus	Rough or smooth	Monoclonal antibodies	Special properties
Typhus	R > S	Yes	Proteus and
Spotted fever	R > S	Yes	Legionella
R. bellii	S	?	Cross-reactive
Scrub typhus	None Detected	-	-
Rochalimaea	R & S	Yes	Small amount
Coxiella	Variable	Yes	Phase variation
Ehrlichia	?	?	Small amount?
Wolbachia	S	Yes	Large amount
Cowdria	?	-	-
Neorickettsia	?	-	-
Rickettsiella	?	-	-

classical LPS extraction methods, silver-staining of LPS after polyacrylamide gel electrophoresis (PAGE), and by Western blotting analysis, typhus and spotted fever group rickettsiae [3, 17, 22, 58, 60, 85] (Fig. 2), *Coxiella* [7, 34, 35, 79, 98-101], *Rochalimaea* [40, Dasch, unpublished observations], and *Wolbachia persica* LPS (Fig. 3A) each exhibit unique multiple band patterns and unique serological properties. Differences in LPS structure among closely related species

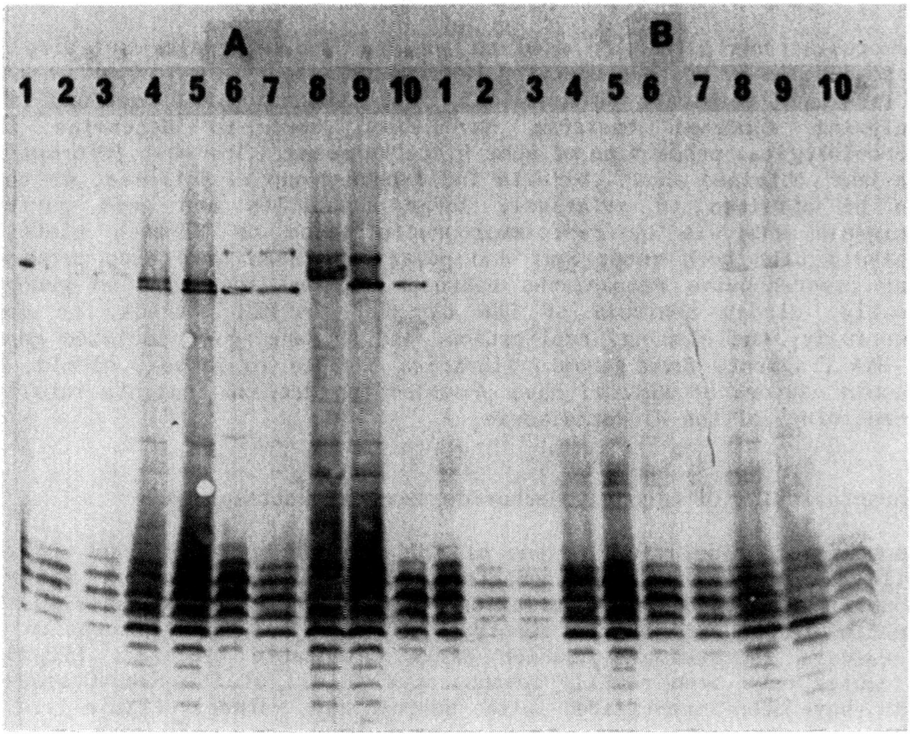

Figure 2. Western blotting analysis of spotted fever group rickettsiae harvested from extracellular culture medium of infected irradiated mouse L cells. Samples (5-15 µg) were separated on 8-16% SDS-PAGE gradient gels after solubilization at room temperature (A) or after boiling (B). After Western blot transfer to nitrocellulose, the antigens were detected with rabbit antiserum to *Rickettsia conorii* simco, horseradish peroxidase-conjugated goat anti-rabbit IgG, and 4-Cl-1-napthol/H2O2 stain. Lanes: 1. *R. conorii* Moroccan, 2. *R. conorii* Casablanca, 3. *R. conorii* Malish, 4. Ethiopian SF2500, 5. Ethiopian SFC84360, 6. Israeli SF CW, 7. Israeli SF CDC, 8. *R. conorii* KTT, 9. *R. conorii* ITT, 10. *R. rickettsii* Price T.

of Rickettsiaceae have also been readily detected. *Rochalimaea vinsonii* and *R. quintana* differ substantially in their autoagglutinability, acting similarly to rough and smooth variants, respectively, of Enterobacteriaceae. Consistent with these differences, the average apparent molecular weight of *R. vinsonii* LPS is much smaller than that of *R. quintana* [19]. Similarly, although both typhus and spotted fever rickettsiae contain relatively large molecules of LPS, the molecular weight distribution is skewed to much lower sizes (Fig. 2) relative to that found for *Rickettsia bellii* [22]. *R. bellii*, in contrast to spotted fever and typhus rickettsiae, appears to lack a crystalline array protein on its surface. This variation in rickettsial LPS type is

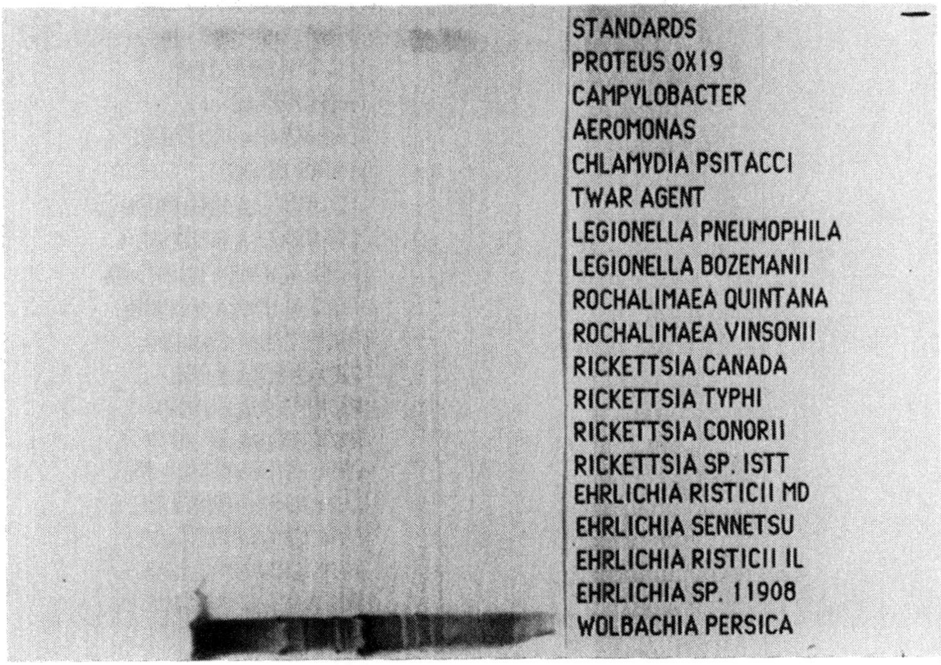

Figure 3. Western blotting analysis of different bacterial species antigens with monoclonal antibodies. Samples (20-40 µg) were solubilized by boiling and analyzed as described in *Figure 2*, except a horseradish peroxidase-conjugated goat anti-mouse IgG was employed in the immunodetection. A. Anti-*Wolbachia persica* LPS monoclonal antibody 134-5C8. B. Anti-*Ehrlichia* 57-58 kDa antigen monoclonal antibody 134-5B1.

strikingly similar to observations made on *Aeromonas salmonicida* and *A. hydrophila*, where the presence of an S-layer protein correlates with the presence of a highly defined size class of LPS [10, 25]. The close structural similarity of typhus and spotted fever LPS to other gram-negative bacteria is further demonstrated by the well-known *Proteus* OX19 and OX2 cross-reactivity (Weil-Felix reaction) of human convalescent sera from infections with typhus and spotted fever group rickettsiae. This cross-reactivity of human rickettsial antisera has more recently been extended to *Legionella bozemanii* and *L. micdadei* and between the two rickettsial groups [58, 60, 68, 97]. Nonetheless, the unique chemistry of each LPS has been demonstrated with polyclonal rabbit sera and monoclonal antibodies and by chemical characterization of both typhus and *Proteus* LPS [3, 60].

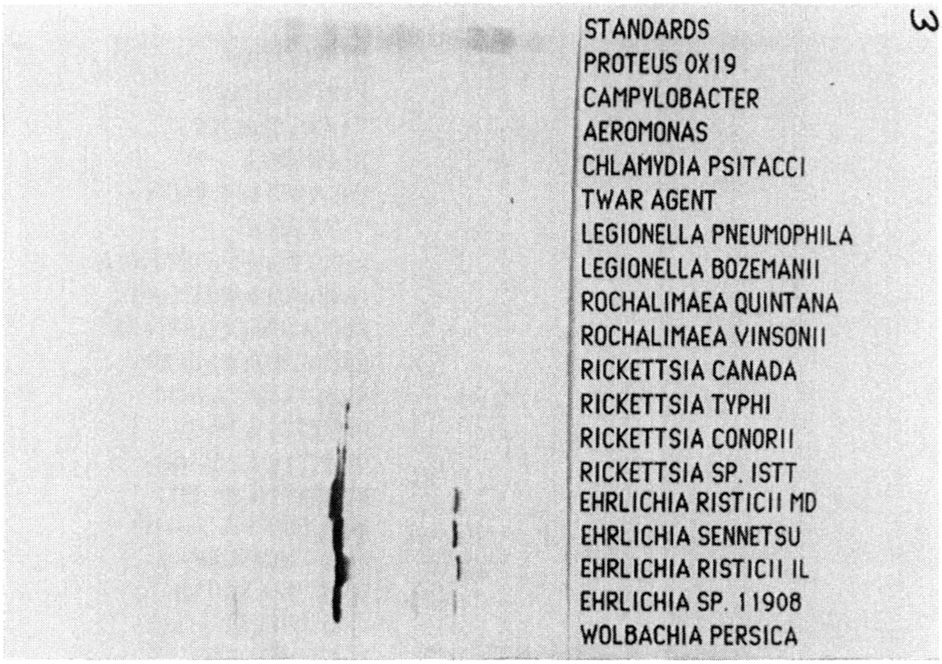

Figure 3. Western blotting analysis of different bacterial species antigens with monoclonal antibodies. Samples (20-40 µg) were solubilized by boiling and analyzed as described in *Figure 2*, except a horseradish peroxidase-conjugated goat anti-mouse IgG was employed in the immunodetection. A. Anti-*Wolbachia persica* LPS monoclonal antibody 134-5C8. B. Anti-*Ehrlichia* 57-58 kDa antigen monoclonal antibody 134-5B1.

The well-known phase variation of *C. burnetii* may also be categorized as a type of smooth to rough LPS variation and even intermediate forms of LPS have been described [1, 34, 35]. Indeed, the purified LPS of *C. burnetii* is the best characterized LPS of the Rickettsiaceae in terms of its chemistry and immunological and biological properties [7, 79].

Since the presence of LPS in *E. risticii* and *E. sennetsu* has not yet been demonstrated unequivocally by Western blotting methods, which readily demonstrate its presence in other Rickettsiaceae (Dasch, unpublished observations), ehrlichial LPS appears to be present only in small amounts, or it may be poorly immunogenic. Unlike the difficulties experienced in detecting LPS in the monocytic ehrlichiae by immunological methods, monoclonal antibodies that recognize *Wolbachia persica* LPS are easily obtained. The very strong reactivity of these antibodies suggests that *W. persica* also contains a large amount of LPS per cell. As shown in Fig. 2A, this LPS appears to be serologically distinct from that present in the other Rickettsiaceae. The lack of suitable methods for obtaining sufficient quantities of bacteria have so far precluded the extension of these studies to other genera of Rickettsiaceae.

Both the presence of LPS and the many parallels in properties of the LPS of Rickettsiaceae to those of the more extensively studied LPS of Enterobacteriaceae are consistent with their common purple eubacterial phylogeny. However, the absence of LPS in *R. tsutsugamushi*, as well as its lack of peptidoglycan [2], suggest that scrub typhus rickettsiae do not belong in the genus *Rickettsia* and may not even belong in the purple eubacteria. On the other hand, it will be very surprising if LPS is not found in the Ehrlichiae and all of the other present species of Rickettsiaceae.

16 S Ribosomal RNA Sequences Of Rickettsiaceae

In recent years, efforts to reconstruct the evolution of prokaryotes by means of direct comparisons of DNA sequences, particularly those of conserved genes encoding the 5S, 16S, and 23S ribosomal RNAs, have been quite fruitful [70, 71, 86, 106]. Among the Rickettsiales, 16S rRNA sequences have been determined for only a few of the diverse species of the Family Rickettsiaceae [87, 89] (Fig. 4). The sequences of each of these species belongs to either the alpha or gamma subdivisions of the purple eubacteria (Class Proteobacteria). The Rickettsiaceae are clearly polyphyletic, as these subdivisions may have begun diverging before the origin of multicellular organisms, and even the relatively close bifurcation of *Rochalimaea* and *Agrobacterium* may have occurred during the time of origin of the plant and animal kingdoms [86].

Notwithstanding the obvious difficulties and hazards involved in attempting to calibrate the temporal rates of evolution of different groups with different mutational rates and selective pressures, these studies provide significant insight into similarities and differences that might not otherwise be apparent. For example, although belonging to distinct lineages and having distinctly different LPS and protein antigens, *Rochalimaea*, typhus and spotted fever rickettsiae, and monocytic *Ehrlichia* all belong to the alpha subdivision of Proteobacteria. *Rochalimaea*, an arthropod-associated bacterium which can be grown free of host cells, was originally thought to be a good biochemical model for the typhus rickettsiae based on a low but specific DNA homology measurement [51]. However, *Rochalimaea* is more closely related to plant-associated bacteria including both the crown-gall, tumor-forming bacterium, *Agrobacterium tumefaciens*, and nitrogen-fixing symbiotic Rhizobiaceae [89]. On the other hand, typhus and spotted fever group rickettsiae, also arthropod-associated but obligate intracellular inhabitants of the eukaryotic cytoplasm, are the closest known bacterial relatives of mitochondria, which are believed to have originated by endosymbiosis. Not surprisingly, the typhus and spotted fever rickettsiae [87] and even *R. bellii* [13] are much more closely related (less than 2% divergence) than *Chlamydia trachomatis* and *C. psittaci* (5% divergence) [88]. Surprisingly, although rickettsiae grow

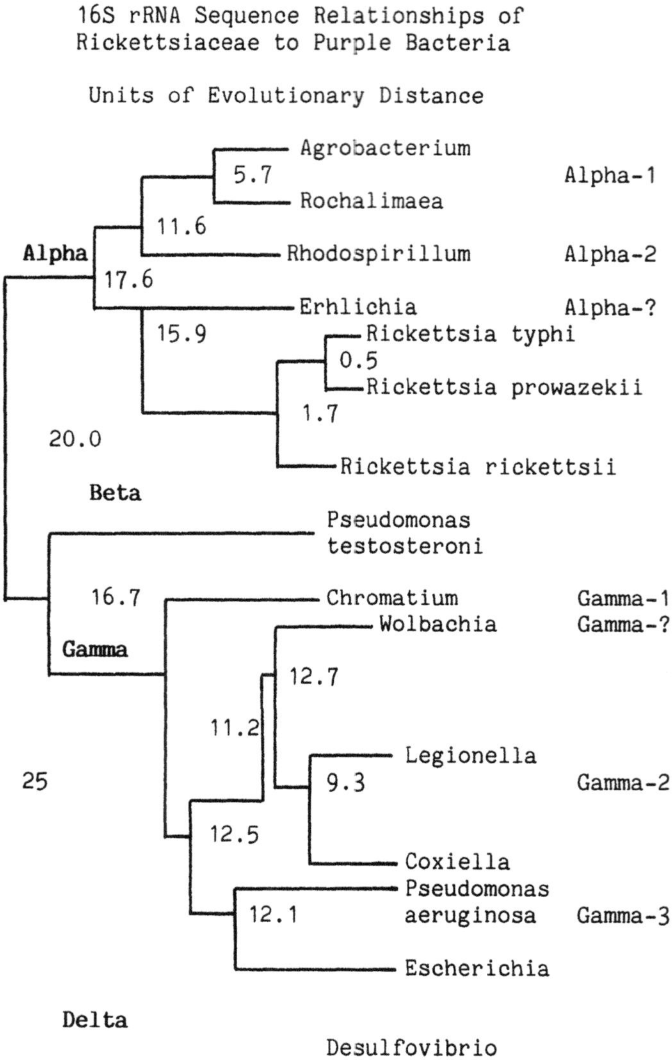

Figure 4. Dendrogram illustrating relationship of Rickettsiaceae whose 16S ribosomal RNA sequences have been determined to the four subdivisions of Proteobacteria. Data adapted from Weisburg et al., 1989 [87] and Woese, 1987 [106]. Units of evolutionary distance on branches are approximate means of values between species on those branches.

freely in the eukaryotic cytoplasm, they are the closest known relatives of the monocytic ehrlichia, *E. risticii*, which grow in a host cell phagosome. Two other intracellular Rickettsiaceae, *W. persica* and *C. burnetii*, are the closest relatives of *Legionella* known, and all belong to the gamma subdivision of Proteobacteria [87]. Although chlamydiae grow in the eukaryotic phagosome, they have a lineage distinctly different from the Proteobacteria [88].

The development of arthropod or host cell associations and obligate parasitism of eukaryotic cytoplasm, phagosome or phagolysosome has obviously arisen many times in evolution. Such associations with vectors or intracellular host cell membranes can be a misleading characteristic for taxonomic purposes. On the other hand, the non-glycolytic Rickettsiaceae are all in the alpha subdivision, while glycolytic Rickettsiaceae are all in the gamma subdivision of purple eubacteria. The extension of 16S rRNA sequencing to *R. tsutsugamushi, Cowdria*, granulocytic ehrlichiae, *Neorickettsia, Rickettsiella*, and other wolbachiae is quite desirable and may be expected to offer some additional surprises and insights.

Electrophoretic Analysis Of Antigens Of Rickettsiaceae

A close evolutionary relationship of typhus and spotted fever group rickettsiae had long been suspected from the reciprocal cross-reactivity of polyclonal sera detected by microimmunofluorescence [37]. That many specific protein antigens, as well as lipopolysaccharides, are involved in this cross-reactivity has been demonstrated by radioimmuno-precipitation [29, 104] and Western blotting analysis (Figures 3, 5, 6) [18, 22, 58, 60, 85]. Western blotting offers advantages over radio-immunoprecipitation in that it avoids the necessity for radiolabelling rickettsial antigens, difficulties in solubilizing some antigens, and the frequent problem of coprecipitation of incompletely solubilized antigen complexes. However, the Western blotting procedure may inadvertently destroy certain important conformational or multisubunit-dependent epitopes. Human sera from patients infected with either the typhus or spotted fever groups of rickettsiae contain anti-LPS antibodies that cross-react with typhus, spotted fever, Proteus, and Legionella lipopolysaccharides. The cross-reactive antibodies are largely IgM [58, 60, 68]. In contrast, hyperimmune rabbit sera commonly have only typhus or spotted fever group specific reactivity (Fig. 2). Consequently, one can use sera from the other group to detect specific protein antigens without having them obscured with the broadly banding LPS reactivity (compare Fig. 2, 5). The Western blots obtained in this manner have permitted us to identify the major protein antigens (120 and 130-180 kDa, 110, 70, and 70-85, 60, 28, and 17 kDa) that are present in both typhus and spotted fever rickettsiae.

The large species-specific protein antigens (SPAs) of 120 and 130-180 kDa, and the 70-85-kDa bands have been particularly valuable for examining species and strain variation of typhus and spotted fever rickettsiae (Fig. 5) [11, 17, 22]. The SPAs are heat-modifiable proteins which are unusually sensitive to temperature changes. The SPAs undergo heat modifiability at 56°C before treatment with SDS and 40°C after treatment with SDS and prior to electrophoresis [17, 21, 85] (Fig. 5). All typhus and spotted fever group monoclonal antibodies that neutralize mouse rickettsial toxicity appear to react with heat-sensitive determinants and many are species-specific [59, 85, 94]. However, some of these antibodies are also cross-reactive and not all

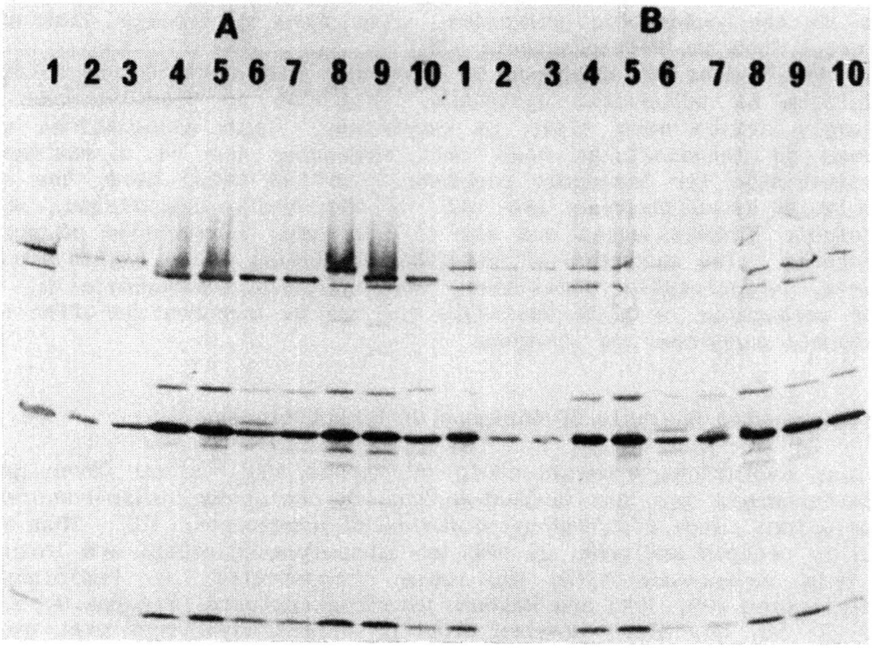

Figure 5. Western blotting analysis of spotted fever group rickettsiae harvested from extracellular culture medium of infected irradiated mouse L cells. Samples (5-15 µg) were separated on 8-16% SDS-PAGE gradient gels following solubilization at room temperature (A) or after boiling (B). After Western blot transfer to nitrocellulose, the antigens were detected with rabbit antiserum to *Rickettsia typhi*, horseradish peroxidase-conjugated goat anti-rabbit IgG, and 4-Cl-1-napthol/H2O2 stain. Lanes: 1. *R. conorii* Moroccan, 2. *R. conorii* Casablanca, 3. *R. conorii* Malish, 4. Ethiopian SF2500, 5. Ethiopian SFC84360, 6. Israeli SF CW, 7. Israeli SF CDC, 8. *R. conorii* KTT, 9. *R. conorii* ITT, 10. *R. rickettsii* Price T.

antibodies recognizing heat-labile SPA epitopes are toxin-neutralizing. Furthermore, a large number of both specific and cross-reactive heat-insensitive epitopes are also present on these large antigens [59, 94]. With the exception of the 28-kDa antigen, either rat or mouse monoclonal antibodies have been obtained against LPS and each of the major protein antigens of typhus rickettsiae recognized by human or rabbit sera (Dasch, unpublished data). Monoclonal antibodies against only the two types of SPA and LPS have been described for the spotted fever group rickettsiae [85].

The well-known antigenic variation of scrub typhus rickettsiae has been studied extensively by analysis of whole cells and subfractions on Coomassie blue-stained gels and by Western blotting analysis with rabbit

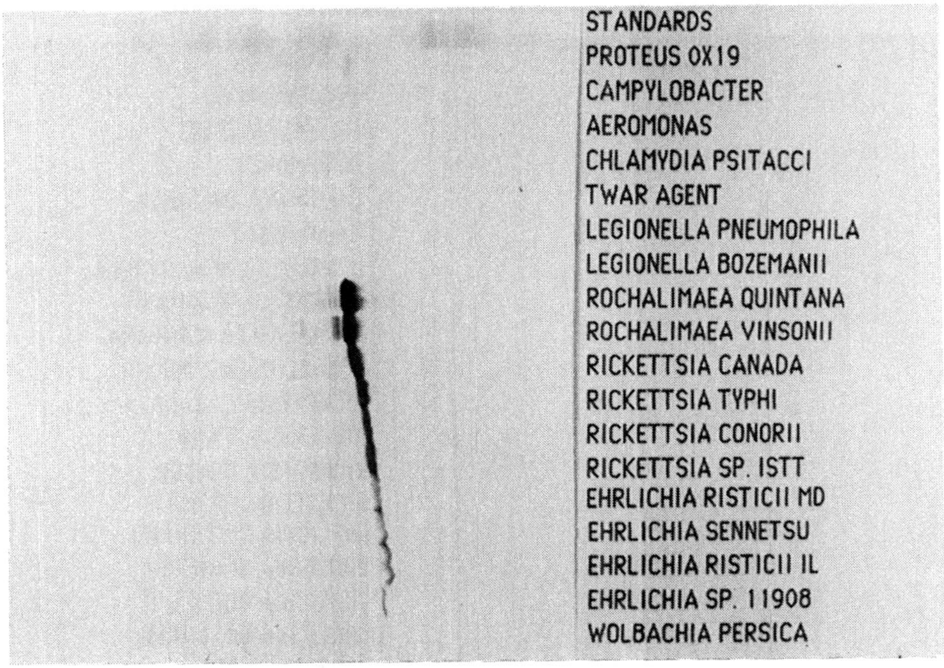

Figure 6. Western blotting analysis of different bacterial species antigens with monoclonal antibodies. Samples (20-40 µg) were solubilized by boiling and analyzed as described in *Figure 2*, except a horseradish peroxidase-conjugated goat anti-mouse IgG was employed in the immunodetection. A. Anti-*Rochalimaea quintana* 60-kDa antigen monoclonal antibody G56-5D2.2. B. Anti-*Mycobacterium leprae* 60-kDa antigen monoclonal antibody IIH9.

and human immune sera and with specific monoclonal antibodies [36, 53, 54, 76, 82]. New strain types have been identified in Japan by using these techniques. The 54-57-kDa major envelope protein of the Karp, Kato, and Gilliam strains has been shown to contain both strain-specific and group-reactive epitopes [36]. Only the 54-57- and 110-kDa antigens were found to exhibit strain heterogeneity in electrophoretic mobility,

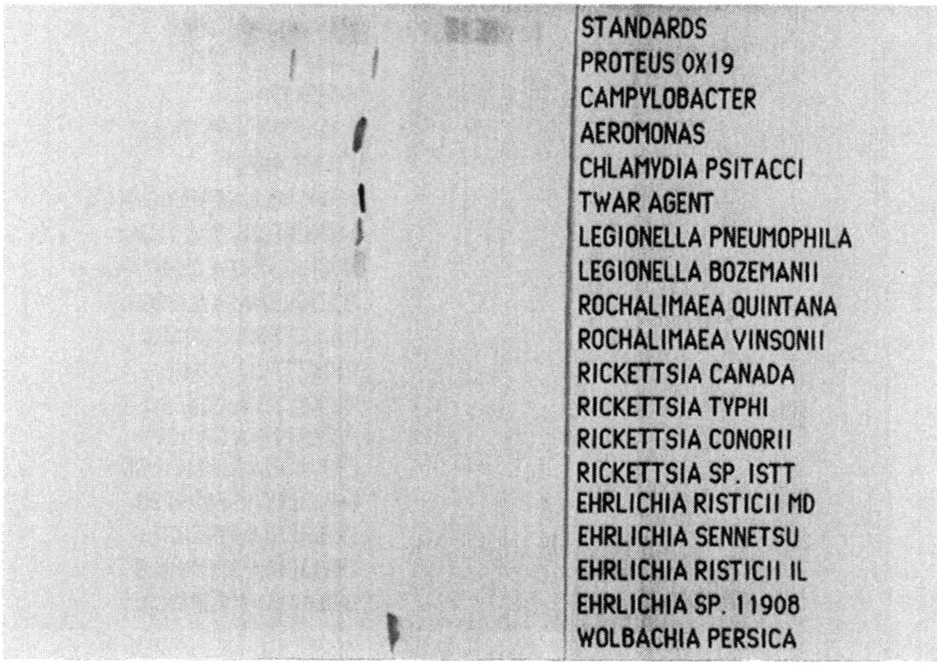

Figure 6. Western blotting analysis of different bacterial species antigens with monoclonal antibodies. Samples (20-40 μg) were solubilized by boiling and analyzed as described in *Figure 2*, except a horseradish peroxidase-conjugated goat anti-mouse IgG was employed in the immunodetection. A. Anti-*Rochalimaea quintana* 60-kDa antigen monoclonal antibody G56-5D2.2. B. Anti-*Mycobacterium leprae* 60-kDa antigen monoclonal antibody IIH9.

while the 21-, 48-, 50-, 59-, 73-, and 150-kDa proteins appeared to be relatively invariant by using Western blot analysis with rabbit antibodies that had been affinity-purified against each of eight cloned Karp strain recombinant antigen fragments [53]. In each case the sera reacted similarly to Karp, Kato, and Gilliam proteins, demonstrating that all shared some epitopes with the cloned Karp antigen fragments.

However, with the exception of the 72-kDa antigen, for each of the other seven antigens, restriction length polymorphisms were detected among Karp, Kato, and Gilliam genomes by using the recombinant Karp antigen gene fragments as probes. In addition, with nine other low-passage human isolates of scrub typhus, 8/9 reacted with 47-, 56-, or 72-kDa antibody; 4/9 reacted with 110-kDa antibody; and 9/9 reacted with 58-kDa antibody [53]. Consequently, although a large number of protein epitopes appear to be highly conserved, antigenic strain heterogeneity in *R. tsutsugamushi* appears to be due to alterations in at least two surface antigens, the 54-57- and 110-kDa variable proteins.

Several studies identifying the protein antigens of *E. risticii* by Western blotting have been done [27, 28, 63]. Nine proteins of 110-, 86-, 70-, 55-, 51-, 49-, 44-, 33-, and 28-kDa protein apparent size can be detected with serum from an infected horse or pony or rabbits. Of these the 51-, 33-, and 28-kDa antigens appeared to be most immunogenic in horses, although the 44-kDa appeared to be both cross-reactive with *E. sennetsu* and strongly reactive later after clinical recovery. A monoclonal antibody recognizing the 28-kDa protein of *E. risticii*, but not *E. sennetsu*, has been used in a competitive ELISA assay for detecting *E. risticii* infections in horses [66]. We have obtained a genus-specific monoclonal antibody which detects a 57-58-kDa protein antigen (that may be the 51-kDa protein described by Dutta et al. [27, 28]) that differs slightly in mobility in two strains of *E. risticii* and cross-reacts with a similar size protein in two strains of *E. sennetsu* (Fig. 2B).

An immunodominant 32-kDa protein antigen has been detected in nine different stocks of *C. ruminantium*, suggesting that it is highly conserved and may be useful as serodiagnostic antigen [42]. The 32-kDa protein does not appear to share epitopes with *E. phagocytophila*, unlike other *Cowdria* antigens. Several other immunogenic polypeptides (200-, 75-, 54-, 44-, 40- and 25- kDa) were detected by Western blotting with goat and mouse antisera.

Immune responses of animals after infection by phase I *C. burnetii* notably produce antibodies against the highly immunogenic surface proteins, followed by the poorly immunogenic LPS [102]. The elicitation of antibodies specific for surface proteins occurs first for the phase II cell, secondly for the phase I cell, and last for the LPS of the phase I cell. This same profile occurs in humans after infection by phase I *C. burnetii* [Williams and Marrie, unpublished results]. Chronic Q fever in humans elicits significant antibody levels to the phase I LPS, which may be diagnostic for the presentation of chronic disease [Williams and Marrie, unpublished results]. In animal models, significant antibody levels to LPS can be induced by immunization with inactivated phase I whole cells [7, 34, 35, 50, 79, 98-101, 103]. A phase I LPS-specific monoclonal antibody has been obtained [99]. Three antigenic groups of phase I LPS variants among acute and chronic strains of *C. burnetii* have been detected with silver staining of LPS or by Western blotting with rabbit anti-phase I LPS antiserum [34, 35]. However, infection of guinea pigs with phase I cells of the acute Nine Mile strain, the Nine Mile/Crazy variant (or CB9MI514) [2], and the goat abortion strain (purported chronic endocarditis strain), Priscilla, elicited similar immune responses and very similar cross-protective responses [50]. Although much as has been described for analysis of typhus and spotted fever antigens (Fig. 2, 5), it is still necessary to either prepare monoclonal antibodies or a serum lacking reactivity to the LPS for one or the other to identify the immunoreactive protein antigens. By Western blotting, rabbit anti-phase II sera detects proteinase K sensitive antigens of 65-, 28-29-, 20-, 16-, and 14-kDa, which are also absent in purified LPS fractions [34, 35]. By Western blotting, guinea pig immune responses to infection with the acute isolate Nine Mile and chronic Priscilla strain were directed against identical 14-, 24-, and 44-kDa antigens in each strain [50]. By radioimmuno-precipitation (RIP) with mouse sera, antigens of 200-, 86-, 48-, 27-, 20.5-, 12.5- and 10.5-kDa were detected with phase I antiserum, while only the 200-, 48-, 27-, and 20.5-kDa antigens were precipitated with phase II antiserum. By Western blotting, mouse sera reacted primarily with 86-, 60-, and 28-kDa antigens [101]. A phase II-specific epitope of a 29.5-kDa protein has also been detected with a monoclonal antibody by RIP but not by Western blots [99]. Although this 29.5-kDa protein was present in both phase I and phase II cells, the phase II-specific epitope was "unmasked" as a result of truncating the phase I LPS [99]. The relationship between these protein antigens will require the development of monoclonals or monospecific polyclonal antibodies against purified or individually cloned and expressed protein antigens in *Escherichia coli* [98].

The only common antigen identified among the Rickettsiaceae so far is the bacterial common protein antigen, which is found in Archaebacteria, spirochetes, chlamydiae, cyanobacteria, gram-positive bacteria, purple eubacteria, and both chloroplasts (rubisco-binding protein), and mitochondria (P1 protein) [26, 39, 41, 67, 78, 108]. These proteins are all members of the highly conserved 58-65-kDa heat-shock proteins (Hsp 60 protein family), which are homologous to the 60-kDa GroEL protein of *E. coli*. Among the rickettsiaceae, the presence of Hsp 60 protein antigens has been demonstrated for all of the typhus and spotted rickettsiae, *R. vinsonii* and *R. quintana, E. risticii*; and *E. sennetsu, W. persica*, (Fig. 5, 6), [19] *C. burnetii* [84], and *R. tsutsugamushi* [73]. Although the classical heat or stress-responsiveness of these proteins has only been demonstrated for *C. burnetii* [80], it is likely that the Hsp 60 proteins of the Rickettsiaceae will soon be shown to have important functions in the assembly of oligomeric proteins (chaperonin function) as well as in the turnover of denatured or aberrant proteins, particularly those generated under stressful physiological conditions, as has been shown for other members of the Hsp 60 family.

Genus-specific anti-Hsp 60 monoclonal antibodies have been obtained for *Ehrlichia, Rochalimaea*, and *Rickettsia* (typhus and spotted fever groups only). Broadly reactive monoclonal antibodies have also defined subgroupings of strains [19]. One anti-*Rochalimaea* monoclonal antibody reacted strongly with all Rickettsiaceae, which are members of the alpha subdivision of purple eubacteria; it reacted very weakly with *Proteus* and *Campylobacter*, but it did not react with any other species (Fig. 6A). An anti-*Mycobacterium leprae* monoclonal antibody was reactive to gamma subdivision purple eubacteria like *C. burnetii* (not shown), *Wolbachia, Legionella, Proteus, Aeromonas*, and to the chlamydiae, which are a distinct branch of eubacteria based on 16S rRNA sequencing, but not to *Campylobacter* or to alpha subdivision Rickettsiaceae (Figure 6B). This observation is quite consistent with the view, based on 16S ribosomal RNA sequences, that *Campylobacter* belongs to a previously undefined branch of eubacteria quite distinct from the spirochetes, chlamydiae, gram-positive bacteria, and purple eubacteria [81].

Although *R. tsutsugamushi* contains a protein antigen that reacts weakly with a variety of polyclonal sera to different Hsp 60 proteins, it does not react with a number of monoclonal antibodies that are broadly reactive against a number of Hsp 60 proteins [19, 73]. This suggests that it too may belong to a previously undefined branch of eubacteria.

Several monoclonal antibodies against *M. leprae*, including II H-9, as well as a polyclonal serum against Chinese hamster mitochondrion protein P1, have been used to demonstrate the immunological cross-reactivity between mammalian and bacterial Hsp 60 proteins [26]. The similarity in the mammalian mitochondrial proteins and bacterial proteins raises the possibility of the involvement of pathogenic bacteria in autoimmune diseases such as rheumatoid arthritis. It is not known whether certain species of Rickettsiaceae have antigens with strong similarity to conserved host antigens like the mitochondrial P1 proteins or whether having such shared determinants would increase the probability of their inducing such undesired host responses.

Cloning And Characterization Of Protein Antigen Genes Of Rickettsiaceae

With the exceptions of the species-specific serotype protein antigens of typhus and spotted fever rickettsiae [11, 15-18, 44, 48], the 56-kDa antigen of *R. tsutsugamushi* [54], the 60-kDa antigens of *Rochalimaea* and typhus rickettsiae [19], and the 29.5-kDa P1 antigen of *C. burnetii* [98], relatively little is known about the biochemistry of individual protein antigens of the Rickettsiaceae [7, 36, 79, 85, 94] because of the daunting task of obtaining sufficient material for these analyses. However, the rapid pace of molecular cloning and sequencing of protein antigen genes that can be identified with monoclonal and polyclonal antisera is providing substantial information about these proteins from their deduced amino acid sequences. As the recombinant antigen genes are engineered into overexpression vectors and large amounts of the encoded proteins become available, the detailed analysis of their B- and T-cell epitopes [9, 11, 12], processing [4, 11], and functional properties [80] may become commonplace.

The strong LPS and protein antigenic cross-reactivity, as well as the similarity in 16S rRNA sequences of the typhus and spotted fever groups have been discussed previously. The cloning and sequencing of genes encoding the 17-kDa and SPA proteins of these rickettsiae have provided direct genetic evidence corroborating their close phylogenetic relationship [4-6, 11, 33, 47-49, 55, 61]. Indeed many of the mutations evident in the DNA sequences of these genes resulted in no changes in amino acid sequence or in highly conservative amino acid changes. Interestingly, N-terminal amino acid modifications have been detected for each protein, and the 120-kDa SPAs appear to undergo an unusual 20%

truncation step in the carboxyl end of the protein. The value of the SPAs as subunit protective vaccines for typhus and spotted fever group rickettsiae [9, 16, 18, 47, 49] may be answered definitively in the next 5 years.

Portions of the genes encoding eight of the major antigens of the Karp strain of *R. tsutsugamushi* have been obtained as lambda gt11 clones. Subsequent isolation, subcloning, and sequencing of the entire genes encoding the 47-, 56-, and 58-kDa antigens have been completed [53, 73, 74, C. K. Stover, personal communication]. Although the 56-kDa antigen gene contains conserved regions that can be used to amplify the gene from DNA of the Karp, Kato and Gilliam strains [43], the purified antigens of these strains have amino terminal sequences that share only 74.3% homology [54]. This is consistent with their great variability in electrophoretic mobility and reactivity with monoclonal antibodies [36, 53]. The 47- or 56-kDa antigens do not have any homology with other known bacterial antigens. In contrast, the 58-kDa sequence has a strong homology with other members of the Hsp 60 (GroEL) family of proteins and its gene is present in a common operon with a small protein with strong homology to the Hsp 10 (GroES) protein of *E. coli* [73]. A similar type of operon containing both GroES and GroEL homologues has also been cloned and sequenced in *C. burnetii* [84]. In contrast to the *Coxiella* Hsp 60 sequence, which has the strongest homology to the *E. coli* sequence of known Hsp 60 sequences, the *R. tsutsugamushi* sequence is as different from those of *Coxiella* and *E. coli* as it is from the Hsp 60 sequences of *C. psittaci*, mitochondria, chloroplasts, or the blue-green alga, *Synechococcus* [19, 73]. The unique phylogenetic position of scrub typhus rickettsiae, as deduced from its Hsp60 protein sequence, is consistent with the unique immunological cross-reactivity pattern of this protein with monoclonal antibodies, as described above. In a more recent study [69] employing restriction length polymorphism analysis of PCR-amplified, 58-kDa sequences from different serotypes of *R. tsutsugamushi*, this conserved antigen exhibited an unexpected degree of variability. It is not clear whether this result means that *R. tsutsugamushi* is comprised of a large number of previously unrecognized species or whether this protein is just unusually variable in this species.

In addition to the Hsp 60 protein, the cloning of two other genes encoding immunogenic proteins has been described for *C. burnetii*. One gene encoded a unprocessed lipoprotein (P2) of 28.9 kDa. The processed P2 was predicted to be 27.1 kDa. The amino acid composition of P2 is different from the previously purified P1 of roughly the same size by SDS-PAGE analysis [98]. P1 was present on the surface of Phase I cells while P2 was exposed on Phase II cells. Another gene encoding a protein of 27-kDa has been cloned into the lambda vector EMBL3 [38]. Monospecific sera prepared against the recombinant protein reacted with a 27-kDa protein that was present in all acute and chronic *C. burnetii* strains tested.

A lambda gt11 clone bank has been made for *E. risticii* [28]. Fragments of the 70- and 44-kDa antigen genes were obtained as fusion peptides with beta-galactosidase, while the 55-kDa antigen was expressed from its own promoter. Although no genes encoding proteins have been obtained, a lambda gt11 clone bank of *C. ruminantium* DNA has been made and used to select clones useful for detecting *Cowdria* DNA [105].

In addition to studies with specific cloned antigen genes, random genetic fragments have been used extensively as probes of the genetic variation of typhus [61, 62] and spotted fever [32, 57, 61] rickettsiae, as well as both the plasmids and genome of *C. burnetii* [46, 65, 83]. Although the rickettsial RFLP detected have been remarkably consistent, with conclusions based on serology, biological properties, and Western blotting analyses, they have reinforced the present taxonomic arrangements and demonstrated that the diversity of rickettsial species is of a lower magnitude than that found for free-living bacterial species [32]. In contrast, these studies have defined six genetic groups of *C. burnetii* which had not been previously recognized [46]. Heterogeneity in the genome size of different *Rickettsiella* species has also been demonstrated by pulse-field gel electrophoresis [31].

Conclusions

While significant progress has been made in understanding the antigenic properties and phylogenetic relationships of selected species of the Rickettsiaceae in the last 5 years, a number of species has received very minimal attention. For some of these species, the lack of analysis may be due to their relatively low importance as causes of human or animal diseases. However, in most cases, the agents are biohazards or extremely expensive to investigate. These difficulties are compounded further by the lack of deposited culture strains for many species, by the lack of continuous culture systems for their routine production, and by poorly understood associations with their host cells which make their purification difficult. However, the advent of sophisticated microchemical procedures, the availability of monoclonal antibodies, and particularly, the powerful tools of recombinant DNA research, have made it possible to overcome these obstacles.

For many of the Rickettsiaceae, LPS is a very important immunogen. However, many details of their chemistry and practically all aspects of their biosynthesis are not known. Indeed, even the existence or importance of LPS as immune modulator in the Ehrlichiae has received no attention as yet. Furthermore, it is not known whether the glycosyltransferases and other enzymes required for their biosynthesis are regulated in a coordinate fashion nor whether they are present in a regulon that might be susceptible to cloning as a complex. Studies of these aspects of LPS of the Rickettsiaceae should proceed as rapidly in the next few years as our understanding of the chemistry of *Coxiella* LPS has in the last decade.

Although many protein antigens have been identified in the different genera of Rickettsiaceae by both radioimmunoprecipitation and Western blotting, only a few of these antigens have been cloned and their entire sequence obtained. It is likely that homologues to heat-shock proteins other than the Hsp 60 family will also be found as major antigens of the Rickettsiaceae as has been found for *Mycobacterium*. Efforts to gain a detailed understanding of the major protein antigens of each species of Rickettsiaceae will require investigation of their biosynthesis, processing, translocation, posttranslational modification by the bacteria or their host cells, and particularly, their function. The overexpression of these antigens in a variety of host systems should permit the development of an entirely new generation of diagnostic reagents and vaccines. Furthermore, access to large quantities of these proteins will permit us to dissect the way in which the humoral and cell-mediated arms of the immune system recognize these antigens.

Lastly, the limited information we have obtained on the Hsp 60 proteins and 16S ribosomal RNA genes is in remarkable concordance with a number of longer-held observations on the relationships of these species. We now have clear genetic evidence that the Rickettsiaceae include a number of phylogenetically unrelated species. The unique characteristics of the scrub typhus rickettsiae make it very difficult to retain them in the genus *Rickettsia* with the closely related typhus and spotted fever group rickettsiae. Growth in a membrane-enclosed host vacuole is a very poor taxonomic characteristic. Parallels in the fatty acid metabolism, LPS, and environmental stability of *Legionella, Coxiella*, and *Wolbachia* appear worth exploring. Finally, it appears that the properties of *Rochalimaea, Ehrlichia*, and *Rickettsia* should be related more to members of the alpha subdivision organisms of purple eubacteria than to the Enterobacteriaceae, which are presently used as paradigms.

Acknowledgements

The work described in this article was done in our laboratories and supported by the Naval Medical Research and Development Command, Department of the Navy, Research Project 3M161102.BS13.AK.111 and the United States Army Medical Research Institute of Infectious Diseases.

Literature Cited

1. **Amano, K.-I., A. Tamura, N. Ohashi, H. Urakami, S. Kaya, and K. Fukushi.** 1987. Deficiency of peptidoglycan and lipopolysaccharide components in *Rickettsia tsutsugamushi*. *Infect. Immun.* **55**:2290-2292.
2. **Amano, K.-I., J. C. Williams, S. R. Missler, and V. N. Reinhold.** 1987. Structure and biological relationship of *Coxiella burnetii* lipopolysaccharides. J. Biol. Chem. **262**:4740-4747.
3. **Amano, K.-I., J. C. Williams, and G. A. Dasch.** 1990. Lipopolysaccharides of *Rickettsia typhi* and *Rickettsia prowazekii*: relationship between contents of quinovosamine and Weil-Felix reaction. In Preparation.
4. **Anderson, B. E., B. R. Baumstark, and W. J. Bellini.** 1988. Expression of the gene encoding the 17-kilodalton antigen from *Rickettsia rickettsii*: transcription and posttranslational modification. *J. Bacteriol.* **170**:4493-4500.
5. **Anderson, B. E., R. L. Regnery, G. M. Carlone, T. Tzianabos, J. E. McDade, Z. Y. Fu, and W. J. Bellini.** 1987. Sequence analysis of

the 17-kilodalton-antigen gene from *Rickettsia rickettsii*. *J. Bacteriol.* **169**:2385-2390.

6. **Anderson, B. E., and T. Tzianabos.** 1989. Comparative sequence analysis of a genus-common rickettsial antigen gene. *J. Bacteriol.* **171**:5199-5201.
7. **Baca, O.** 1988. Surface antigens of *Coxiella burnetii*, p. 127-134. *In* D. H. Walker (ed.), Biology of Rickettsial Diseases, Vol. II. CRC Press, Boca Raton, FL.
8. **Bezuidenhout, J. D.** 1987. The present state of *Cowdria ruminantium* cultivation in cell lines. *Onderstepoort J. Vet. Res.* **54**:205-210.
9. **Carl, M., and G. A. Dasch.** 1989. The importance of the crystalline surface layer protein antigens of rickettsiae in T-cell immunity, p. 81-91, *In* M. Feldmann, R. N. Maini, and J. Woody ed.), T-cell activation in health and disease. *J. Autoimmunity 2(Suppl.)*.
10. **Chart, H., D. H. Shaw, E. E. Ishiguro, and T. J. Trust.** 1984. Structural and immunochemical homogeneity of *Aeromonas salmonicida* lipopolysaccharide. *J. Bacteriol.* **158**:16-22.
11. **Ching, W-M., G. A. Dasch, M. Carl, and M. E. Dobson.** 1990. Structural analysis of the 120 kDa serotype protein antigens (SPAs) of typhus rickettsiae. Comparison with the properties of other S-layer proteins. *Ann. N. Y. Acad. Sci.* In Press.
12. **Churilla, A., W-M. Ching, G. A. Dasch, and M. Carl.** 1990. Human T lymphocyte recognition of CNBr fragments of the surface protein (SPA) of *Rickettsia typhi*. *Ann. N. Y. Acad. Sci.* In Press.
13. **Clark, J., C. Pretzman, P. Perlman, and P. Fuerst.** 1989. The 16S rRNA gene sequence of *Rickettsia bellii* and the evolution of *Rickettsia*. *J. Bacteriol.* Submitted.
14. **Cole, A. I., M. Ristic, G. E. Lewis, Jr., and G. Rapmund.** 1985. Continuous propagation of *Ehrlichia sennetsu* in murine macrophage cell cultures. *Am. J. Trop. Med. Hyg.* **34**:774-780.
15. **Dasch, G. A.** 1981. Isolation of species-specific protein antigens of *Rickettsia typhi* and *Rickettsia prowazekii* for immunodiagnosis and immunoprophylaxis. *J. Clin. Microbiol.* **14**:333-341.
16. **Dasch, G. A., and A. L. Bourgeois.** 1981. Antigens of the typhus group of rickettsiae: importance of the species-specific surface protein antigens in eliciting immunity, p. 61-70, *In* W. Burgdorfer and R. L. Anacker (ed.), Rickettsiae and rickettsial diseases. Academic Press, New York.
17. **Dasch, G. A., J. P. Burans, M. E. Dobson, R. I. Jaffe, and W. G. Sewell.** 1985. Distinctive properties of components of the cell envelope of typhus group rickettsiae, p. 54-61, *In* J. Kazar (ed.), Rickettsiae and rickettsial diseases. Publishing House of the Slovak Academy of Sciences, Bratislava.
18. **Dasch, G. A., J. P. Burans, M. E. Dobson, F. M. Rollwagen, and J. Misiti.** 1984. Approaches to subunit vaccines against the typhus rickettsiae, *Rickettsia typhi* and *R. prowazekii*, p. 251-256, *In* D. Schlessinger (ed.), *Microbiology 1984*. American Society for Microbiology, Washington, D.C.
19. **Dasch, G. A., W.-M. Ching, P. Y. Kim, H. Pham, C. K. Stover, E. V. Oaks, M. E. Dobson, and E. Weiss.** 1990. A structural and immunological comparison of rickettsial Hsp 60 proteins with those of other species. *Ann. N. Y. Acad. Sci.* In Press.

20. **Dasch, G. A., S. Halle, and A. L. Bourgeois.** 1979. Sensitive microplate enzyme-linked immunosorbent assay for detection of antibodies against the scrub typhus rickettsia, *Rickettsia tsutsugamushi*. *J. Clin. Microbiol.* **9**:38-48.
21. **Dasch, G. A., J. R. Samms, and J. C. Williams.** 1981. Partial purification and characterization of the major species-specific protein antigens of *Rickettsia typhi* and *Rickettsia prowazekii* identified by rocket immuno-electrophoresis. *Infect. Immun.* **31**:276-288.
22. **Dasch, G. A., W. G. Sewell, W. Burgdorfer, and R. Grays.** 1990. Rapid immunotyping of the spotted fever group of rickettsiae: evidence for significant antigenic diversity in strains from the Mediterranean, African and Asian subcontinent. *Curr. Microbiol.* Submitted.
23. **Dasch, G. A., and E. Weiss.** 1977. Characterization of the Madrid E strain of *Rickettsia prowazekii* purified by Renografin density gradient centrifugation. *Infect. Immun.* **15**:280-286.
24. **Dasch, G. A., and E. Weiss.** 1978. Factors affecting the viability of *Rickettsia tsutsugamushi* purified from yolk sacs and L cells, p. 115-127, *In* J. Kazar, R. A. Ormsbee, and I. N. Tarasevich (ed), Rickettsiae and rickettsial diseases. VEDA, Slovak Academy of Science, Bratislava, Czechoslovakia.
25. **Dooley, J. S. G., R. Lallier, and T. J. Trust.** 1986. Surface antigens of virulent strains of *Aeromonas hydrophila*. *Vet. Immunol. Immunopathol.* **12**:339-344.
26. **Dudani, A. K., and R. S. Gupta.** 1989. Immunological characterization of a human homolog of the 65-kilodalton mycobacterial antigen. *Infect. Immun.* **57**:2786-2793.
27. **Dutta, S. K., B. L. Mattingly, and B. Shankarappa.** 1989. Antibody response to *Ehrlichia risticii* and antibody reactivity to the component antigens in horses with induced Potomac horse fever. *Infect. Immun.* **57**:2959-2962.
28. **Dutta, S. K., B. Shankarappa, and B. Mattingly.** 1990. Characterization and antigenicity of recombinant major antigens of *Ehrlichia risticii*. *Ann. N. Y. Acad. Sci.* In Press.
29. **Feng, H. M., C. Kirkman, and D. H. Walker.** 1986. Radioimmunoprecipitation of [^{35}S]methionine-radiolabeled proteins of *Rickettsia conorii* and *Rickettsia rickettsii*. *J. Infect. Dis.* **154**:717-721.
30. **Frank, D. W., T. C. McGuire, J. R. Gorham, and W. C. Davis.** 1974. Cultivation of two species of *Neorickettsia* in canine monocytes. *J. Infect. Dis.* **129**:247-262.
31. **Frutos, R., M. Pages, M. Bellis, G. Roizes, and M. Bergoin.** 1989. Pulsed-field gel electrophoresis determination of the genome size of obligate intracellular bacteria belonging to the genera *Chlamydia*, *Rickettsiella*, and *Porochlamydia*. *J. Bacteriol.* **171**:4511-4513.
32. **Fuerst, P.** 1990. Molecular genetics of populations: the spotted fever group. *Ann. N. Y. Acad. Sci.* In Press.
33. **Gilmore, R. D., Jr.** 1990. Characterization of the 120-KD surface protein gene of *Rickettsia rickettsii* (R strain). *Ann. N. Y. Acad. Sci.* In Press.

34. **Hackstadt, T.** 1986. Antigenic variation in the phase I lipopolysaccharide of *Coxiella burnetii* isolates. *Infect. Immun.* **52**:337-340.
35. **Hackstadt, T., M. G. Peacock, P. J. Hitchcock, and R. L. Cole.** 1985. Lipopolysaccharide variation in *Coxiella burnetii*: intrastrain heterogeneity in structure and antigenicity. *Infect. Immun.* **48**:359-365.
36. **Hanson, B.** 1988. Role of composition of *Rickettsia tsutsugamushi* in immunity to scrub typhus, p. 111-125, *In* D. H. Walker (ed.), Biology of rickettsial diseases, Vol. II. CRC Press, Boca Raton, FL.
37. **Hechemy, K. E., D. Raoult, J. Fox, Y. Han, L. B. Elliott, and J. Rawlings.** 1989. Cross-reaction of immune sera from patients with rickettsial diseases. *J. Med. Microbiol.* **29**:199-202.
38. **Hendrix, L. R., J. E. Samuel, and L. P. Mallavia.** 1990. Identification and cloning of a ~27KD *Coxiella burnetii* immunoreactive protein. *Ann. N. Y. Acad. Sci.* In Press.
39. **Hindersson, P., C. S. Petersen, N. S. Pedersen, N. Hoiby, and N. H. Axelsen.** 1984. Immunological cross-reaction between antigen Tp-4 of *Treponema pallidum* and an antigen common to a wide range of bacteria. *Acta Path. Microbiol. Immunol. Scand.* B **92**:183-188.
40. **Hollingdale, M. R., J. W. Vinson, and J. E. Herrmann.** 1980. Immunochemical and biological properties of the outer membrane-associated lipopolysaccharide and protein of *Rochalimaea quintana*. *J. Infect. Dis.* **141**:672-678.
41. **Jindal, S., A. K. Dudani, B. Singh, C. B. Harley, and R. S. Gupta.** 1989. Primary structure of a human mitochondrial protein homologous to the bacterial and plant chaperonins and to the 65-kilodalton mycobacterial antigen. *Mol. Cell. Biol.* **9**:2279-2283.
42. **Jongejan, F., and M. J. C. Thielemans.** 1989. Identification of an immunodominant antigenically conserved 32-kilodalton protein from *Cowdria ruminantium*. *Infect. Immun.* **57**:3243-3246.
43. **Kelly, D. J., D. Marana, C. Stover, E. Oaks, and M. Carl.** 1990. Detection of *Rickettsia tsutsugamushi* by gene amplification using polymerase chain reaction. *Ann. N. Y. Acad. Sci.* In Press.
44. **Li, H., and D. H. Walker.** 1990. Biological characterization of major polypeptides on the rickettsial surface. *Ann. N. Y. Acad. Sci.* In Press.
45. **Logan, L. L., T. C. Whyard, J. C. Quintero, and C. A. Mebus.** 1987. The development of *Cowdria ruminantium* in neutrophils. *Onderstepoort J. Vet. Res.* **54**:197-204.
46. **Mallavia, L. P., J. E. Samuel, and M. E. Frazier.** 1990. The genetics of *Coxiella burnetii*, etiologic agent of Q fever and chronic endocarditis, pp. xxxx, *In* J. C. Williams (ed.), The biology of *Coxiella burnetii* the etiologic bacterial pathogen of Q fever. CRC Press, Boca Raton, Fl.
47. **McDonald, G. A., R. L. Anacker, and K. Garjian.** 1987. Cloned gene of *Rickettsia rickettsii* surface antigen: candidate vaccine for Rocky Mountain spotted fever. *Science* **235**:83-85.
48. **McDonald, G. A., R. L. Anacker, and R. E. Mann.** 1988. Extraction of protective components of *Rickettsia rickettsii* with n-octyl-

[beta]-D-glucopyranoside. *Rev. Infect. Dis.* **10**(supplement 2):S382-S385.

49. **McDonald, G. A., R. L. Anacker, R. E. Mann, and L. J. Milch.** 1988. Protection of guinea pigs from experimental Rocky Mountain spotted fever with a cloned antigen of *Rickettsia rickettsii*. *J. Infect. Dis.* **158**:228-231.
50. **Moos, A., and T. Hackstadt.** 1987. Comparative virulence of intra- and interstrain lipopolysaccharide variants of *Coxiella burnetii* in the guinea pig model. *Infect. Immun.* **55**:1144-1150.
51. **Myers, W. F., and C. L. Wisseman, Jr.** 1980. Genetic relatedness among the typhus group of rickettsiae. *Int. J. Syst. Bacteriol.* **30**:143-150.
52. **Nyindo, M. B. A., M. Ristic, D. L. Huxsoll, and A. R. Smith.** 1971. Tropical canine pancytopenia: in vitro cultivation of the causative agent--*Ehrlichia canis*. *Am. J. Vet. Res.* **32**:1651-1658.
53. **Oaks, E. V., R. M. Rice, D. J. Kelly, and C. K. Stover.** 1989. Antigenic and genetic relatedness of eight *Rickettsia tsutsugamushi* antigens. *Infect. Immun.* **57**:3116-3122.
54. **Ohashi, N., A. Tamura, M. Ohta, and K. Hayashi.** 1989. Purification and partial characterization of a type-specific antigen of *Rickettsia tsutsugamushi*. *Infect. Immun.* **57**:1427-1431.
55. **Policastro, P. F., B. E. Anderson, and G. A. McDonald.** 1990. Structure and expression of the gene encoding the 155kD surface antigen of *Rickettsia rickettsii*. *Ann. N. Y. Acad. Sci.* In Press.
56. **Pretzman, C. I., Y. Rikihisa, D. Ralph, J. C. Gordon, and S. Bech-Nielsen.** 1987. Enzyme-linked immunosorbent assay for Potomac horse fever disease. *J. Clin. Microbiol.* **25**:31-36.
57. **Ralph, D., C. Pretzman, N. Daugherty, and K. Poetter.** 1990. Genetic relationships among the members of the family rickettsiaceae as shown by DNA restriction fragment polymorphism analysis. *Ann. N. Y. Acad. Sci.* In Press.
58. **Raoult, D., and G. A. Dasch.** 1989. Line blot and Western blot immunoassays for diagnosis of Mediterranean spotted fever. *J. Clin. Microbiol.* **27**:2073-2079.
59. **Raoult, D., and G. A. Dasch.** 1989. The line blot: an immunoassay for monoclonal and other antibodies. Its application to the serotyping of gram-negative bacteria. *J. Immunol. Meth.* In Press.
60. **Raoult, D., Dasch, G. A., and Hussong, D.** 1990. Lipopolysaccharide cross-reactions among species of typhus and spotted fever group rickettsiae, *Proteus* and *Legionella*, by sera from patients with Mediterranean spotted fever. *Infect. Immun.* Submitted.
61. **Regnery, R. L.** 1990. Use of DNA probes for differentiation of spotted fever group and other rickettsiae. *Ann. N. Y. Acad. Sci.* In Press.
62. **Regnery, R. L., Z. Y. Fu, and C. L. Spruill.** 1986. Flying squirrel-associated *Rickettsia prowazekii* (epidemic typhus rickettsiae) characterized by a specific DNA fragment produced by restriction endonuclease digestion. *J. Clin. Microbiol.* **23**:189-191.
63. **Rikihisa, Y., C. I. Pretzman, G. C. Johnson, S. M. Reed, S. Yamamoto, and F. Andrews.** 1988. Clinical, histopathological, and

immunological responses of ponies to *Ehrlichia sennetsu* and subsequent *Ehrlichia risticii* challenge. *Infect. Immun.* **56**:2960-2966.
64. **Ristic, M.** 1986. Pertinent characteristics of leukocytic rickettsiae of humans and animals, p. 182-187, *In* L. Leive (ed.), *Microbiology--1986.* American Society for Microbiology, Washington, D.C.
65. **Samuel, J. E., M. E. Frazier, and L. P. Mallavia.** 1985. Correlation of plasmid type and disease caused by *Coxiella burnetii. Infect. Immun.* **49**:775-779.
66. **Shankarappa, B., S. K. Dutta, J. Sanusi, and B. L. Mattingly.** 1989. Monoclonal antibody-mediated, immunodiagnostic competitive enzyme-linked immunosorbent assay for equine monocytic ehrlichiosis. *J. Clin. Microbiol.* **27**:24-28.
67. **Shinnick, T. M., M. H. Vodkin, and J. C. Williams.** 1988. The *Mycobacterium tuberculosis* 65-kilodalton antigen is a heat shock protein which corresponds to common antigen and to the *Escherichia coli* GroEL protein. *Infect. Immun.* **56**:446-451.
68. **Sompolinsky, D., I. Boldur, R. A. Goldwasser, H. Kahana, R. Kazak, A. Keysary, and A. Pik.** 1986. Serological cross-reactions between *Rickettsia typhi, Proteus vulgaris* OX19 and *Legionella bozemanii* in a series of febrile patients. *Isr. J. Med. Sci.* **22**:745-752.
69. **Spruill, C., and R. L. Regnery.** 1990. Analysis of *Rickettsia tsutsugamushi* amplified DNA that codes for antigenic and metabolic gene products. *Ann. N. Y. Acad. Sci.* In Press.
70. **Stackebrandt, E.** 1988. Phylogenetic relationships vs. phenotypic diversity: how to achieve a phylogenetic classification system of the eubacteria. *Can. J. Microbiol.* **34**:552-556.
71. **Stackebrandt, E., R. G. E. Murray, and H. G. Truper.** 1988. *Proteobacteria* classis nov., a name for the phylogenetic taxon that includes the "purple bacteria and their relatives." *Int. J. Syst. Bacteriol.* **38**:321-325.
72. **Stephenson, E. H., and J. V. Osterman.** 1980. Somatic cell hybrids of canine peritoneal macrophages and SV40-transformed human cells: derivation, characterization, and infection with *Ehrlichia canis. Am. J. Vet. Res.* **41**:234-240.
73. **Stover, C. K., E. V. Oaks, D. Marana, and G. A. Dasch.** 1990. The 58 kDa immuno-dominant antigen of *Rickettsia tsutsugamushi* is a homologue of the 60 kDa heat shock protein family: molecular cloning and sequence analysis of the regulon encoding the Stp11 and Sta58 proteins. *J. Bacteriol.* Submitted.
74. **Stover, C. K., M. H. Vodkin, and E. V. Oaks.** 1987. Use of conversion adaptors to clone antigen genes in lambda gt11. *Anal. Biochem.* **163**:398-407.
75. **Suitor, E. C., Jr.** 1964. Propagation of *Rickettsiella popilliae* (Dutky and Gooden) Philip and *Rickettsiella melolonthae* (Krieg) Philip in cell cultures. *J. Insect. Pathol.* **6**:31-40.
76. **Tamura, A., N. Ohashi, H. Urakami, K. Takahashi, and M. Oganagi.** 1985. Analysis of polypeptide composition and antigenic components of *Rickettsia tsutsugamushi* by polyacrylamide gel electrophoresis and immunoblotting. *Infect. Immun.* **48**:671-675.
77. **Tamura, A., H. Urakami, and T. Tsuruhara.** 1982. Purification of

Rickettsia tsutsugamushi by Percoll density gradient centrifugation. *Microbiol. Immunol.* **26**:321-328.

78. **Thole, J. E. R., P. Hindersson, J. de Bruyn, F. Cremers, J. van der Zee, H. de Cock, J. Tommassen, W. van Eden, and J. D. A. van Embden.** 1988. Antigenic relatedness of a strongly immunogenic 65kDA mycobacterial protein antigen with a similarly sized ubiquitous bacterial common antigen. *Microb. Pathogen.* **4**:71-83.
79. **Thompson, H. A.** 1988. Relationship of the physiology and composition of *Coxiella burnetii* to the *Coxiella*-host cell interaction, p. 51-78. In D. H. Walker (ed.), Biology of rickettsial diseases, Vol. II. CRC Press, Boca Raton, FL.
80. **Thompson, H. A., C. Bolt, T. A. Hoover, and J. C. Williams.** 1990. Induction of heat shock proteins in *Coxiella burnetii*. *Ann. N. Y. Acad. Sci.* In Press.
81. **Thompson, L. M., III, R. M. Smibert, J. L. Johnson, and N. R. Krieg.** 1988. Phylogenetic study of the genus *Campylobacter*. *Int. J. Syst. Bacteriol.* **38**:190-200.
82. **Urakami, H., N. Ohashi, T. Tsuruhara, and A. Tamura.** 1986. Characterization of polypeptides in *Rickettsia tsutsugamushi*: effect of preparative conditions on migration of polypeptides in polyacrylamide gel electrophoresis. *Infect.Immun.* **51**:948-952.
83. **Vodkin, M. H., and J. C. Williams.** 1986. Genetic heterogeneity among isolates of *Coxiella burnetii*. *J. Gen. Microbiol.* **132**:455-463.
84. **Vodkin, M. H., and J. C. Williams.** 1988. A heat shock operon in *Coxiella burnetii* produces a major antigen homologous to a protein in both mycobacteria and *Escherichia coli*. *J. Bacteriol.* **170**:1227-1234.
85. **Walker, D. H.** 1988. Role of the composition of rickettsiae in rickettsial immunity: typhus and spotted fever groups, p. 101-109, *In* D. H. Walker (ed.), Biology of rickettsial diseases, Vol. II. CRC Press, Boca Raton, FL.
86. **Weisburg, W. G.** 1989. Polyphyletic origin of bacterial parasites, p. 1-15, *In* J. W. Moulder (ed.), Intracellular parasitism. CRC Press, Inc., Boca Raton, FL.
87. **Weisburg, W. G., M. E. Dobson, J. E. Samuel, G. A. Dasch, L. P. Mallavia, O. Baca, L. Mandelco, J. E. Sechrest, E. Weiss, and C. R. Woese.** 1989. Phylogenetic diversity of the rickettsiae. *J. Bacteriol.* **171**:4202-4206.
88. **Weisburg, W. G., T. P. Hatch, and C. R. Woese.** 1986. Eubacterial origin of chlamydiae. *J. Bacteriol.* **167**:570-574.
89. **Weisburg, W. G., C. R. Woese, M. E. Dobson, and E. Weiss.** 1985. A common origin of rickettsiae and certain plant pathogens. *Science* **230**:556-558.
90. **Weiss, E.** 1981. The family Rickettsiaceae: human pathogens, p. 2137-2160, *In* M. P. Starr, H. Stolp, H. G. Truper, A. Balows, and H. G. Schlegel (ed.), The prokaryotes. A handbook on habitats, isolation, and identification of bacteria. Vol. II. Springer-Verlag, New York.
91. **Weiss, E., J. C. Coolbaugh, and J. C. Williams.** 1975. Separation of viable *Rickettsia typhi* from yolk sac and L cell host components by Renografin density gradient centrifugation. *Appl. Microbiol.* **30**:456-463.

92. **Weiss, E., G. A. Dasch, Y.-H. Kang, and H. N. Westfall.** 1988. Substrate utilization by *Ehrlichia sennetsu* and *Ehrlichia risticii* separated from host constituents by Renografin gradient centrifugation. *J. Bacteriol.* **170**:5012-5017.
93. **Weiss, E., G. A. Dasch, Y.-H. Kang, and J. C. Williams.** 1990. Comparison of properties of isolated ehrlichiae and scrub typhus rickettsiae. *Ann. N. Y. Acad. Sci.* In Press.
94. **Weiss, E., Dobson, M. E., and Dasch, G. A.** 1987. Biochemistry of rickettsiae: recent advances. *Acta Virol.* **31**:271-286.
95. **Weiss, E., and J. W. Moulder.** 1984. The rickettsias and chlamydias, p. 687-739, *In* N. R. Krieg and J. G. Holt (ed.), Bergey's manual of Systematic Bacteriology, vol. 1. The Williams and Wilkins Co. Baltimore, MD.
96. **Weiss, E., J. C. Williams, G. A. Dasch, and Y.-H. Kang.** 1989. Energy metabolism of monocytic *Ehrlichia*. *Proc. Natl. Acad. Sci. USA* **86**:1674-1678.
97. **Westfall, H., N., R. A. Goldwasser, E. Weiss, and D. Hussong.** 1986. Prevalence of antibodies to *Legionella* species in a series of patients in Israel. *Isr. J. Med. Sci.* **22**:131-138.
98. **Williams, J. C., T. A. Hoover, D. M. Waag, N. Banerjee-Bhatnagar, C. R. Bolt, and G. H. Scott.** 1990. Antigenic structure of *Coxiella burnetii*: a comparison of lipopolysaccharide and protein antigens as vaccines against Q fever. *Ann. N. Y. Acad. Sci.* In Press.
99. **Williams, J. C., M. R. Johnston, M. G. Peacock, L. A. Thomas, S. Stewart, and J. L. Portis.** 1984. Monoclonal antibodies distinguish phase variants of *Coxiella burnetii*. *Infect. Immun.* **43**:421-428.
100. **Williams, J. C., M. G. Peacock, and T. F. McCaul.** 1981. Immunological and biological characterization of *Coxiella burnetii*, phase I and phase II, separated from host components. *Infect. Immun.* **32**:840-851.
101. **Williams, J. C., and S. Stewart.** 1984. Identification of immunogenic proteins of *Coxiella burnetii* phase variants, p. 257-262, *In* L. Leive and D. Schlessinger (ed.), *Microbiology 1984*. American Society for Microbiology, Washington, D.C.
102. **Williams, J. C., L. A. Thomas, and M. G. Peacock.** 1986. Humoral immune response to Q fever: enzyme-linked immunosorbent assay antibody response to *Coxiella burnetii* in experimentally infected guinea pigs. J. Clin. Microbiol. **24**:935-939.
103. **Williams, J. C., L. A. Thomas, and M. G. Peacock.** 1986. Identification of phase-specific antigenic fraction of *Coxiella burnetii* by enzyme-linked immunosorbent assay. J. Clin. Microbiol. **24**:929-934.
104. **Williams, J. C., D. H. Walker, M. G. Peacock, and S. T. Stewart.** 1986. Humoral immune response to Rocky Mountain spotted fever in experimentally infected guinea pigs: immunoprecipitation of lactoperoxidase ^{125}I-labeled proteins and detection of soluble antigens of *Rickettsia rickettsii*. *Infect. Immun.* **52**:120-127.
105. **Wilkins, S. C., and R. E. Ambrosio.** 1989. The isolation of nucleic acid sequences specific for *Cowdria ruminantium*. *Onderstepoort J. Vet. Res.* **56**:127-129.

106. **Woese, C. R.** 1987. Bacterial evolution. *Microbiol. Rev.* **51**:221-271.
107. **Woldehiwet, Z., and G. R. Scott.** 1982. In vitro propagation of *Cytoecetes phagocytophila*, the causative agent of tick-borne fever. *Vet. Microbiol.* **7**:127-133.
108. **Young, D. B., J. Ivanyi, H. K. Cox, and J. R. Lamb.** 1987. The 64 kDa antigen of mycobacteria--a common bacterial protein? *Immunol. Today* **8**:215-219.

5. BIOLOGICAL PROPERTIES OF THE GENUS *EHRLICHIA*: SUBSTRATE UTILIZATION AND ENERGY METABOLISM

E. WEISS, Ph.D.
G. A. DASCH, Ph.D.
J. C. Williams, Ph.D.
Y-H. KANG, Ph.D.

Abstract

Our increased awareness of *Ehrlichia* as pathogens of humans and animals has prompted us to investigate their biological properties. This study was initiated with the Miyayama strain of *E. sennetsu* and the Illinois and Maryland strains of *E. risticii*. The ehrlichiae, harvested from heavily infected P388D$_1$ mouse macrophage cells, were separated from host constituents by procedures that included mechanical disruption of the cells, digestion with trypsin and DNAase, and separation by either Renografin or Percoll density gradient centrifugation. Such preparations were used immediately or after storage in a liquid N_2 chest. Of the substrates tested, the ehrlichiae utilized glutamine most rapidly, glutamate to a slight extent, and glucose not at all. The most favorable suspending medium, containing sucrose and potassium phosphate, provided some osmotic protection and was moderately alkaline. The ATP levels of the ehrlichial preparations were tested by the firefly luminescence test. The initial low ATP levels of such preparations were increased significantly by incubation for 1 hour at 34°C with glutamine. Such levels were reduced somewhat by the addition of atractyloside and, to a greater extent, by the addition of 2,4-dinitrophenol. Control preparations derived from uninfected P388D$_1$ cells did not display the activities demonstrated with the ehrlichial preparations. We conclude that, with respect to metabolic activities, *Ehrlichia* more closely resemble *Rickettsia* than *Chlamydia*.

Introduction

In 1981 Miodrag Ristic and one of us (E. W.) were working on the new edition of Bergey's Manual [6] in association with Jim Moulder. Dr. Ristic was interested in many genera, including the genus *Ehrlichia*, while my interest was primarily in the tribe *Rickettsieae*. I was making good progress, but I got stuck when I was confronted with the species *Rickettsia sennetsu* that just did not fit in the genus *Rickettsia*. Finally, I wrote to Dr. Ristic and referred the *sennetsu* agent to him, hoping he could find a place for it in the genus *Ehrlichia*. Dr. Ristic replied immediately accepting the sennetsu agent. He included in his letter two pre-prints [5, 11] from his laboratory, which made it very clear that the *sennetsu* agent was indeed an ehrlichia.

J. C. Williams and I. Kakoma (eds.), Ehrlichiosis, 59–67.

Thus, the bulk of the data reported in this and related chapters is based on the pioneering work of Ristic and his associates. They have been very kind to us, sent us three strains of *Ehrlichia* and have encouraged us to proceed as we did.

On the topic of important contributions that have made our study possible, we would like to mention the work of Marianna Bovarnick, who initiated the study of the molecular biology of the rickettsiae. In 1949 Bovarnick and John Snyder [3] demonstrated for the first time that typhus rickettsiae respire in the presence of glutamate. Subsequently, Bovarnick [1] showed that rickettsiae form ATP, when incubated with glutamate. In this first study, she used an ingenious indicator system for the measurement of ATP. It consisted of glucose, which rickettsiae do not utilize, plus ADP, hexokinase, and inorganic phosphate. Any ATP that was generated led to the formation of glucose-6-phosphate which was measured by the reduction of exogenous NADP in the presence of glucose-6-phosphate dehydrogenase. In subsequent studies with Allen [2], she measured ATP by means of the firefly luminescence system.

With respect to metabolism, ehrlichiae utilize exogenously supplied substrates very much like rickettsiae. However, there is a slight difference [14, 15], in that the chief substrate of ehrlichiae is glutamine and not glutamate. We speculate that the difference in the metabolism of these two molecules lies in the fact that glutamate is a highly charged molecule and that some cells do not readily transport it. In contrast, glutamine is transported more efficiently, but is rapidly deaminated to glutamate and catabolized via the citric acid cycle. This hypothesis is strengthened by our observation [15] that the low level of glutamate catabolism of *Ehrlichia* is somewhat enhanced by exogenous glutamine. Many bacteria utilize glutamate better than glutamine since the deamination step is not necessary. *Ehrlichia* differ from the intracellular bacterium *Wolbachia persica* in that they do not utilize glucose [16] and from chlamydiae in that they do not utilize glucose-6-phosphate [8, 18].

Methods and Results

Our first series of experiments [14, 15] were done with ehrlichiae purified by Renografin density gradient centrifugation. *Ehrlichia risticii* cells purified by this method are apparently free of host components. There was a great variety in morphology (e.g., large and small, different electron density etc.). In contrast to preparations of rickettsiae prepared by the identical procedure, a number of membranes of host origin were retained in the ehrlichial preparations and, in some cases, the host membranes enclosed a typical morula structure.

More recently, we purified the ehrlichiae by the Percoll density gradient procedure [17, Dasch *et al.*, in preparation], which has been shown to be particularly useful for the purification of *Rickettsia tsutsugamushi* [12]. In our experiments, prior to gradient separation, the infected cell homogenates were treated first with trypsin, then with DNAase, and finally with DNAase plus trypsin inhibitor. Three fractions were obtained after Percoll gradient centrifugation. The bottom fraction was the most highly purified. Although the latter fraction did not look too different from the cells purified by Renografin, the cells were more metabolically active. The intermediate fraction contained some host material including empty shells, but it also had a fair number of ehrlichiae, possibly a subpopulation of the ehrlichiae retained in the bottom fraction. The top fraction consisted of a wide assortment of host material and empty shell, but undoubtedly a few ehrlichia cells were still trapped. This fraction was discarded, or kept as a "negative" control.

The advantage of using Percoll purified ehrlichiae was clearly shown in our tests of catabolism of added substrates and in our studies of ATP formation after incubation with glutamine. For example, in our previous experiments with Renografin purified material, we frequently observed moderate amounts of CO_2, in the presence of glucose-6-phosphate plus nicotinamide adenine dinucleotide phosphate (NADP). The significance of this phenomenon was hard to explain. When the cells were purified by Percoll, it became quite clear that the dehydrogenases involved were host enzymes. The host-derived dehydrogenose activity was greatly reduced by proteolytic enzyme treatment and was practically eliminated by Percoll fractionation [Dasch *et al.*, in preparation].

We have shown [17] that ehrlichiae, carefully purified in the cold ($4^{o}C$) by Renografin or Percoll gradients, contain small amounts of ATP. Upon incubation at 34°C for 1 hour without substrate, ATP was catabolized while in the presence of glutamine its concentration increased. Although the two purification procedures involved more than one variable and the results must be interpreted with caution, it is clear that the concentrations of ATP before and after incubation with glutamine were substantially higher in the Percoll-purified cells. Furthermore, the actions of atractyloside and 2,4-dinitrophenol (DNP) (which were expected to be non-inhibitory and inhibitory, respectively, of ATP formation in bacteria) were more clearly shown with the Percoll purified preparations, suggesting, in this case, also greater freedom from host enzymes (Fig. 1).

An ehrlichia that is of particular interest to us is strain 11908, which is most likely a strain of *E. sennetsu*. It was isolated by Adeinka Cole, whose promising work was unfortunately truncated at a very early age. Cynthia Holland was kind enough to send us some of his reports, from which we will try to reconstruct the isolation of this strain. *Ehrlichia sennetsu*, although very similar in biological properties to *E. risticii* and related to *E. canis*, was believed to be a human disease confined to a small region of Japan. More recently, extensive surveys of sera from Malaysia and the Philippines, to which Cole greatly contributed, indicated a high level of seroprevalence among patients suffering from fevers of unknown origin [9]. Cole selected eight whole blood samples from those sent to him by George Lewis from the Kuala Lumpur United States Army Medical Research Unit. The specimens were first inoculated into the peritoneal cavities of mice and passaged into the $P388D_1$, mouse macrophage cell line. In only one of these serial passages, with specimen 11908, was an agent first seen after four consecutive tissue culture passages. By the 9th passage, growth was quite abundant. The culture that we received from the University of Illinois was subsequently grown in our laboratory in $P388D_1$ cells and purified by Percoll gradient centrifugation. Cole

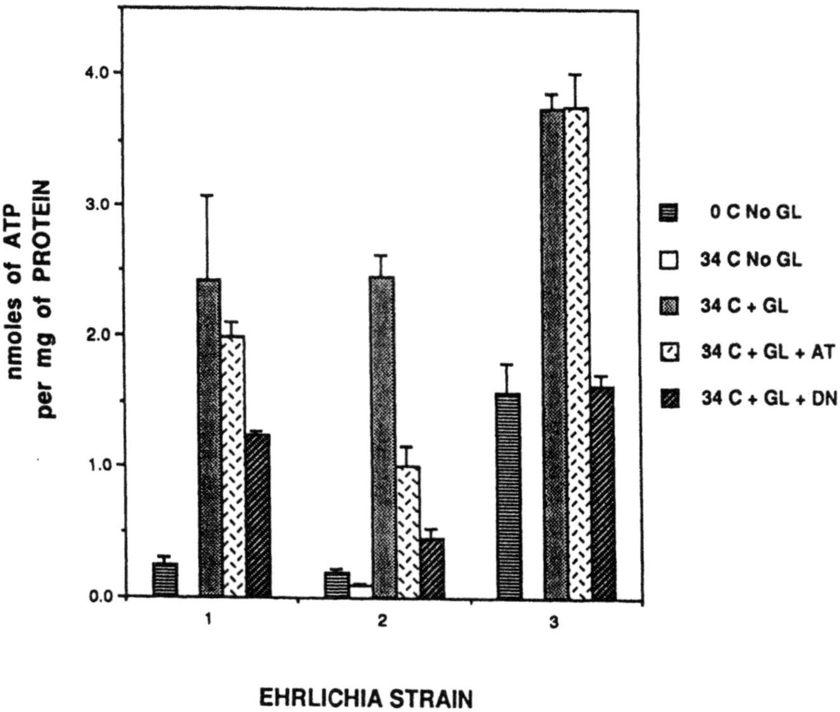

Figure 1. Influence of various factors on the ATP content of *Ehrlichia*, purified either by Renografin or Percoll gradient centrifugation. The three strains, described in a previous publication [15], were as follows: 1. *E. sennetsu*, purified by Renografin; 2. *E. risticii*, Maryland strain, purified by Renografin; 3. *E. risticii*, Illinois strain, purified by Percoll. The cells were maintained in ice water or incubated for 1 hour at 34°C, as indicated. The abbreviations used are as follows: GL, glutamine; AT, atractyloside (an inhibitor of adenine nucleotide translocase in mitrochcondria, but not in bacteria); DN, 2,4-dinitrophenol (an inhibitor of oxidative phosphorylation in both mitochondria and bacteria). For further details, see Ref. [17].

greatly contributed to the establishment of the $P388D_1$ cell line as the most useful for the growth of large quantities of ehrlichia cells for biological and antigenic studies [4].

Table 1 illustrates an experiment with *Ehrlichia* strain 11908 in which we proceeded from the homogenized pools to nuclease and protease treatments and separation by Percoll gradient centrifugation. The protein content was greatly reduced from the original material and only about 3% remained in the bottom fraction, which had the most highly purified ehrlichia cells. On the other hand, glutamine catabolism was reduced to a much lesser extent. The specific metabolic activity increased as we proceeded from the homogenized pool to enzyme treatment, and to the bottom fraction. The specific metabolic activity was also reduced in the intermediate and top fractions. Note that a low

TABLE 1. Protein recovery and metabolic activity during Percoll purification of *Ehrlichia* strain 11908.

Step in purification	Protein Percent	Glutamine catabolism[a] Percent	Specific activity[b]
Homogenate	100	100	62
Enzyme treated	21.4	71.2	209
Percoll fractions[c] I	3.1	21.4	428
II	4.4	4.2	60
III	5.2	1.8	12

[a]Measured as nanomoles CO_2 formed from carbons 1-5 of 1 mM glutamine, after 1 hour of incubation at 34°C.
[b]Nanomoles/mg protein.
[c]The fractions tested: I=bottom; II=intermediate; III=top.

concentration of glutamine, 1 mM, was used in this experiment. The specific activity was somewhat higher, about 600 nmoles CO_2/mg protein, when the glutamine concentration was increased to 5 mM. These results are typical of what we have obtained with the other strains of *Ehrlichia*.

TABLE 2. Metabolic activities of the three Percoll fractions following purification of *Ehrlichia* strain 11908.

Substrate[a] (Carbons labeled)	Metabolic activity[b] of fractions Bottom	Intermediate	Top
Glutamine (1-5)	683	139	31
Glutamate (1-5)	91	21	9.8
Glucose (1-6)	35	10.1	3.6
Glucose-6-P (1)	13.4	3.9	2.5
plus NADP	14.2	9.6	17

[a]The molarites of the substrates were as follows: glutamate and glutamine 5 mM; glucose, glucose-6-phosphate, and NADP 1 mM. In addition, since the cells were maintained in 1 mM glutamine during purification and storage and were diluted, but not washed, all tubes contained an additional 0.067 mM glutamine.
[b]Expressed as nmoles/mg protein after 1 hour of incubation at 34°C. Values are the means of triplicate tests. The standard deviations of the triplicate determinations averaged approximately 5% of the means.

However, when we proceeded with other experiments with the 11908 strain, we ran into some serious difficulties. Table 2 illustrates an experiment in which we tested the three Percoll gradient fractions for

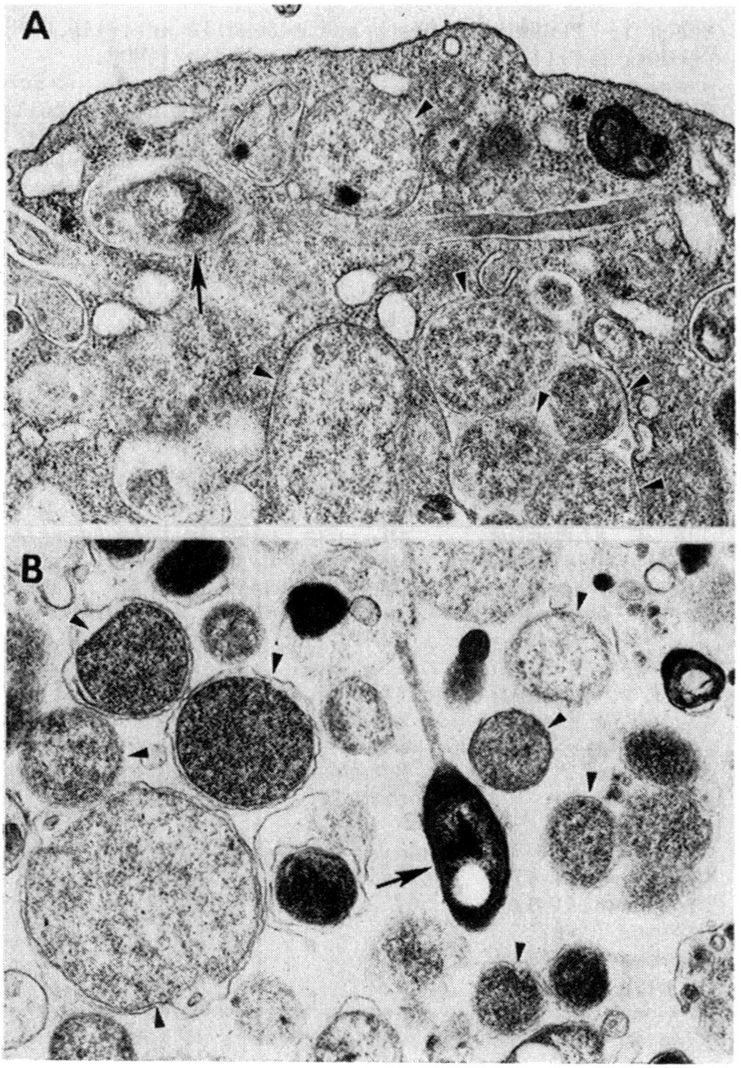

Figure 2. Transmission electron micrographs of *Ehrlichia* strain 11908. Arrowheads point to various types of *Ehrlichia* cells. Arrows point to unidentified contaminant with large appendage. A. Infected $P388D_1$ cell. Magnification, x 32,000. B. Purified preparation, bottom fraction of Percoll gradient. Magnification, x 25,000.

catabolic activity against a number of substrates. The results with glutamine and glutamate were as we expected, and CO_2 production from glucose-6-phosphate in the presence of NADP, although a bit higher than we like to see, was not too much out of line. However, when we examined the catabolism of glucose and glucose-6-phosphate in the absence of cofactor, the levels of CO_2 production were definitely higher than what we have seen before. Most disturbing is the fact that the specific activity was highest in the bottom fraction. We suspected bacterial contamination, despite the fact that no bacteria grew on blood plates or thioglycollate broth and Giemsa and acridine orange slides indicated that the pools were loaded with ehrlichiae. We examined electron micrographs of infected cells and purified material (Fig. 2). There we found among numerous typical ehrlichial cells an intracellular bacterium, not larger than an ehrlichia, but morphologically quite different. The bacterium had a very large appendage, seen in longitudinal sections. The outer surface was too thick for a gram-negative bacterium, but sometimes an outer membrane bilayer can be seen. The microorganisms stain gram-positive, provided that ethyl alcohol and not a mixture of ethyl alcohol and acetone is used for destaining. A vacuole, usually seen, possibly represents a poly-β-hydroxy-butyrate inclusion.

We recently received a fresh seed from Cynthia Holland and repeated this work. No contaminant was detected by electron microscopy and there was no CO_2 production from glucose or glucose-6-phosphate in the bottom fraction. We are convinced now that contamination occurred in our laboratory. We have not identified the contaminant and we are discussing it here for two reasons. Contaminants on rare occasions are quite interesting microorganisms and this one certainly falls into this category. Jim Moulder told us in his excellent review [7] that gram-positive bacteria are very seldom intracellular. Secondly, when working with a non-glycolytic bacterium, a test of glucose metabolism can be a very sensitive method for detecting contamination. The presence of this contaminant does not invalidate our preliminary experiments of glutamine metabolism with ehrlichia cells purified by Percoll gradients. Further work can now be done with our pools free of the contaminant. We are convinced that strain 11908 is a typical *Ehrlichia*, which metabolized glutamine most rapidly of all the substrates tested and derives energy from it.

Conclusion

How do these results compare with those obtained with other intracellular bacteria? We obtained entirely comparable results with *Rickettsia typhi*, except that the ATP levels were higher. To the best of our knowledge, identical experiments have not been carried out with chlamydiae, but there is excellent evidence that the metabolism of chlamydiae does not yield energy and chlamydiae are totally dependent on the host cells for their ATP [8, 18]. Thus, ehrlichiae, with respect to energy metabolism resemble rickettsiae and not chlamydiae.

What do these results mean? They agree with those of Weisburg *et al.*, [13], who examined the 16S rRNA sequences of a number of intracellular bacteria. He and his colleagues showed that ehrlichiae are specifically related to the rickettsiae and not to chlamydiae.

The evolution of bacteria proceeds in very strange ways. Ehrlichiae share many phenotypic characteristics with chlamydiae [10], a location in the host-cell phagosome, and an ability to inhibit phagosome-lysosome fusion, as it has been recently proven by Wells and Rikihisa [19]. Ehrlichiae also have some sort of developmental cycle that superficially resembles that of chlamydiae. However, while the elementary and reticulate bodies can be clearly separated in chlamydiae [8], this has not been done with ehrlichiae.

How do we explain the relatedness between ehrlichiae and rickettsiae? Obviously their microenvironment, ehrlichiae in the phagosome and rickettsiae in the host-cell cytoplasm, is not of paramount importance in evolution. Such differences may be due to just one or two functions. The escape of the rickettsiae from the phagosome is due to a phospholipase [20], which, presumably, is not present in ehrlichiae or acts in a different manner. If rickettsiae, as chlamydiae and ehrlichiae, have a mechanism for preventing phagosome-lysosome fusion, their rapid escape from the phagosome would prevent its detection.

Perhaps in searching for phenotypic clues to explain the evolutionary similarity between ehrlichiae and rickettsiae, we should pay greater attention to their macro-environment. We should be encouraged to search further for possible arthropod vectors for the ehrlichiae, as we are doing for rickettsiae, and examine in greater detail the roles of the smaller mammals, such as the rabbit, mouse, cat, or dog, that might be essential parts of the ecosystems of ehrlichiae or rickettsiae.

Acknowledgements

This work was supported by the Naval Medical Research and Development Command, Department of the Navy, Research Project 3M161102.BS10.AK.111, and the United States Army Medical Research Institute of Infectious Diseases, Department of the Army.

Literature Cited

1. **Bovarnick, M. R.** 1956. Phosphorylation accompanying the oxidation of glutamate by the Madrid E strain of typhus rickettsiae. *J. Biol. Chem.* **220**:353-361.
2. **Bovarnick, M. R., and E. G. Allen.** 1957. Reversible inactivation of the toxicity and hemolytic activity of typhus rickettsiae by starvation. *J. Bacteriol.* **74**:637-645.
3. **Bovarnick, M. R., and J. C. Snyder.** 1949. Respiration of typhus rickettsiae. *J. Exp. Med.* **89**:561-565.
4. **Cole, A. I., M. Ristic, G. E. Lewis, Jr., and G. Rapmund.** 1985. Continuous propagation of *Ehrlichia sennetsu* in murine macrophage cell cultures. *Am. J. Trop. Med. Hyg.* **34**:774-780.
5. **Hoilien, C. A., M. Ristic, D. L. Huxsoll, and G. Rapmund.** 1982. *Rickettsia sennetsu* in human blood monocyte cultures: similarities to the growth cycle of *Ehrlichia canis*. *Infect. Immun.* **35**:314-319.

6. **Krieg, N. R., and J. G. Holt (ed).** 1984. Bergey's manual of systematic bacteriology, vol. 1. The Williams & Wilkins Co., Baltimore.
7. **Moulder, J. W.** 1985. Comparative biology of intracellular parasitism. *Microbiol. Rev.* **49**:298-337.
8. **Moulder, J. W.** 1984. Looking at chlamydiae without looking at their hosts. *ASM News* **50**:353-362.
9. **Rapmund, G.** 1984. Rickettsial diseases of the Far East: new perspectives. *J. Infect. Dis.* **149**:330-338.
10. **Ristic, M.** 1986. Pertinent characteristics of leukocytic rickettsiae of human and animals, p. 182-187. *In* L. Leive (ed.) Microbiology-1986. ASM, Washington, D.C.
11. **Ristic, M., D. L. Huxsoll, N. Tachibana, and G. Rapmund.** 1981. Evidence of serologic relationship between *Ehrlichia canis* and *Rickettsia sennetsu*. *Am. J. Trop. Med. Hyg.* **30**:1324-1328.
12. **Tamura, A., H. Urakami, and T. Tsuruhara.** 1982. Purification of *Rickettsia tsutsugamushi* by Percoll density gradient centrifugation. *Microbiol. Immunol.* **26**:321-328.
13. **Weisburg, W. G., M. E. Dobson, J. E. Samuel, G. A. Dasch, L. P. Mallavia, O. Baca, L. Mandelco, J. E. Sechrest, E. Weiss, and C. R. Woese.** 1989. Phylogenetic diversity of the rickettsiae. *J. Bacteriol.* **171**:4202-4206.
14. **Weiss, E., G. A. Dasch, and Y-H. Kang.** 1985. Glutamine metabolism of *Ehrlichia sennetsu*, p. 38-45. *In* J. Kazar (ed.), Rickettsiae and rickettsial diseases. Slovak Academy of Science, Bratislava, Czechoslovakia.
15. **Weiss, E., G. A. Dasch, Y-H. Kang, and H. N. Westfall.** 1988. Substrate utilization by *Ehrlichia sennetsu* and *Ehrlichia risticii* separated from host contituents by Renografin gradient centrifugation. *J. Bacteriol.* **170**:5012-5017.
16. **Weiss, E., W. F. Myers, E. C. Suitor, Jr., and E. M. Neptune, Jr.** 1982. Respiration of a rickettsialike microorganism, *Wolbachia persica*. *J. Infect. Dis.* **110**:155-164.
17. **Weiss, E., J. C. Williams, G. A. Dasch, and Y-H. Kang.** 1989. Energy metabolism of monocytic *Ehrlichia*. *Proc. Natl. Acad. Sci. USA.* **86**:1674-1678.
18. **Weiss, E. and N. N. Wilson.** 1969. Role of exogeneous adenosine triphosphate in catabolic and synthetic activities of *Chlamydia*. *J. Bacteriol.* **97**:719-724.
19. **Wells, M. Y. and Y. Rikihisa.** 1988. Lack of lysosomal fusion with phagosomes in $P388D_1$ cells: abrogation of inhibition with oxytetracycline. *Infect. Immun.* **56**:3209-3215.
20. **Winkler, H. H., and E. T. Miller.** 1982. Phospholipase A and the interaction of *Rickettsia prowazekii* and mouse fibroblasts (L-929 cells). *Infect. Immun.* **38**:109-113.

6. BIOLOGIC AND PATHOGENIC PROPERTIES OF *EHRLICHIA RISTICII*: THE ETIOLOGIC AGENT OF EQUINE MONOCYTIC EHRLICHIOSIS

CYNTHIA J. HOLLAND, Ph.D.

Abstract

The etiologic agent of the recently recognized disease, equine monocytic ehrlichiosis (EME, synonymous with Potomac horse fever), was isolated in 1984. Antigenic analyses confirmed this microorganism to be a new species of the genus *Ehrlichia*. The agent was subsequently named *Ehrlichia risticii* in honor of Miodrag Ristic for his numerous scientific contributions to the study of rickettsiae and rickettsial diseases. *Ehrlichia risticii* is a gram-negative staining, pleomorphic bacterium, with a preference for growth in monocytes, and ranging in size from 0.4 to 0.75 μm long. The microorganisms occur within vacuoles as single or multiple intracytoplasmic inclusion bodies. *Ehrlichia risticii* has been successfully cultured *in-vitro* by using primary equine and canine blood monocytes as well as the continuous cell lines $P388D_1$ (murine macrophage) and U937 (human histiocyte). L-glutamine is required for growth in tissue culture. The microorganism is strongly inhibited *in-vitro* by antibiotics. Antigenically, *E. risticii* is most closely related to the human pathogen, *E. sennetsu*. Experimentally, dogs, cats, mice, and non-human primates have been shown to be susceptible to infection with *E. risticii*. Clinically, EME is a non-contagious, infectious equine disease often characterized by fever, depression, anorexia, leukopenia, colic, mild to severe diarrhea, and with a mortality rate as high as 30%. Fetal infections may occur. The suspected arthropod vector has not been identified. Equine monocytic ehrlichiosis is widespread, with cases being confirmed in 38 states of the United States, in Canada, and in France. The indirect immunofluorescent antibody test is used for serodiagnosis. Although a newly developed vaccine for prevention of EME has greatly reduced the number of clinical cases, the disease remains a serious threat to the equine industry.

Introduction

Equine monocytic ehrlichiosis (EME), best known as Potomac horse fever (PHF) and occasionally as equine ehrlichial colitis, was first described as a clinical entity affecting horses in Montgomery County, Maryland, in 1979 [34]. Subsequently, other cases were reported in Virginia, Pennsylvania, New Jersey, Ohio, and Idaho.

Typically EME is clinically manifested by any or all of the following: fever, depression, anorexia, distal edema of the limbs, ventral edema, colic, mild to severe diarrhea, and laminitis [15]. Between 1979 and 1984, the mortality rate in affected horses was reported to be as high as 30%. Early studies on EME revealed that the

J. C. Williams and I. Kakoma (eds.), Ehrlichiosis, 68–77.

disease was not contagious [34] but, rather, transmissable only through the inoculation of whole blood derived from acutely infected horses to susceptible horses [13]. Despite early intensive efforts to determine the cause of this devastating disease, the etiologic agent remained evasive. A corona-like virus [12] and several common bacteria and toxins [7], isolated from naturally infected horses, were suspected as the causative agents. However, these agents failed to induce the disease when inoculated into horses. Additional serologic studies with antigens of known equine pathogens also proved unsuccessful in identifying a common disease agent.

A major breakthrough occurred in 1984 when sera, obtained from both naturally and experimentally infected horses, were examined by indirect immunofluorescent antibody (IFA) against three major species of the genus *Ehrlichia*: *E. equi*, the etiologic agent of equine ehrlichiosis; *E. canis*, the etiologic agent of canine ehrlichiosis; and *E. sennetsu*, the etiologic agent of sennetsu fever, a human pathogen, which is believed to be geographically limited to Japan and other regions of Southeast Asia [24]. While none of the sera reacted against *E. equi*, some sera reacted weakly against *E. canis* and all convalescent phase sera reacted relatively strongly against *E. sennetsu* [9, 10]. All preinoculation sera obtained from experimental horses were negative to the above agents. These results indicated that the etiologic agent of EME was a bacterium of the genus *Ehrlichia*. Techniques for the *in-vitro* isolation of *E. canis* [16] and *E. sennetsu* [11] in tissue culture were successfully applied to the isolation of an intracellular bacterium from the peripheral blood monocytes of experimentally infected horses during the acute phase of EME [9]. This finding was subsequently confirmed by other investigators [6, 19] when they independently isolated a bacterium morphologically indistinguishable from the original isolate. This *in-vitro* propagated bacterium consistently induced typical signs of EME in experimentally infected horses, thereby fulfilling Koch's postulates [9]. Based upon results of morphologic, antigenic, and serologic studies, the etiologic agent of EME was confirmed to be a member of the genus *Ehrlichia* [24]. The microorganism was named *E. risticii* in honor of Miodrag Ristic for his valuable contributions to the field of rickettsiae and rickettsial diseases [11].

Biologic Properties of *Ehrlichia risticii*

Ehrlichia risticii is an obligate intracellular bacterium which may be easily cultured *in-vitro* by using primary equine or canine blood monocyte cell cultures [9], the murine macrophage cell line $P388D_1$ [25], or the human histiocyte cell line U937 [19]. Under light microscopy, the bacteria may appear singly, in clusters, or as inclusions (morulae) within the phagosomal vacuole of the host cell (Figure 1). The microorganism stains gram-negative and bluish-purple with Wright-Giemsa stain. Electron microscopy has revealed that the microorganism is contained either singly or multiply within cytoplasmic phagosomal vacuoles (Figure 2). The bacteria exhibit a considerable degree of pleomorphism: round, oval, or elongated, and ranging in size from 0.4 to 0.75 μm in width and from 0.5 to 1.2 μm in length. The microorganism

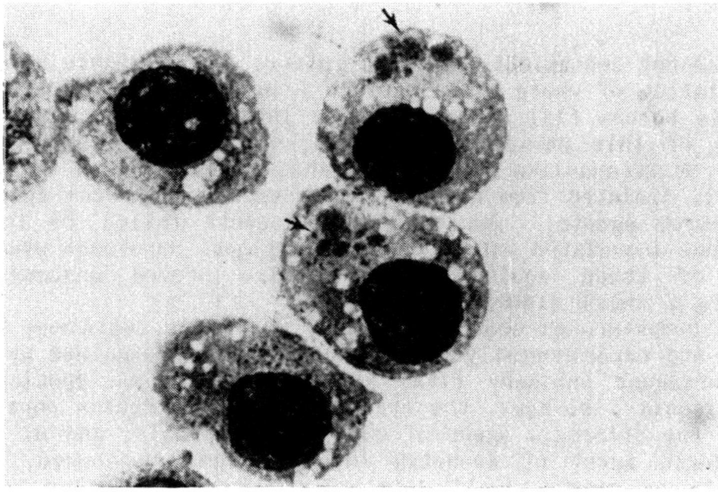

Figure 1. *Ehrlichia risticii* inclusions (arrows) in $P388D_1$ cell cultures. Giemsa stain.

appears to multiply by transverse binary fission, and a development cycle has been suggested by several investigators. Individual bacteria with a highly rippled cell wall are surrounded by a double plasma membrane [11, 31].

Routine culture medium consists of medium 199 (GIBCO) supplemented with 1% L-glutamine and 10% fetal bovine serum (heat-inactivated), adjusted to pH 7.2-7.4 with sodium bicarbonate (5% w/v). Optimal growth in this medium is achieved at 37°C to 38°C under normal atmospheric conditions or in the presence of 5% CO_2, depending on the host cell.

Similar to other ehrlichiae, *E. risticii* preferentially metabolizes L-glutamine *in-vitro* [11, 32] and an acid pH inhibits the metabolism of exogenously supplied substrates [32]. Growth of *E. risticii* is restricted by low concentrations of antibiotics such as penicillin, streptomycin, gentamicin, rifampin, tetracycline, and oxytetracycline with the latter proving to be the most effective [11, 21]. Wells and Rikihisa [33] showed that, by an as yet undetermined mechanism, *E. risticii* is able to inhibit phagosome-lysosome fusion, thereby allowing for its survival within the phagosome of the macrophage. However, when oxytetracycline is added at relatively low concentrations (10 µg/ml) to the culture medium, ehrlichia-containing phagosomes readily fuse with lysosomes, thereby enhancing the destruction of the microorganism.

Utilizing the $P388D_1$ macrophage cell line, a system was established which allowed the continuous *in-vitro* propagation of *E. risticii* [25]. This system has facilitated the production of large quantities of antigen for use in various immunologic studies and in the development of an IFA test for diagnosis and seroepidemiologic studies of EME. Cross-reactivity studies by the IFA test indicate that *E. risticii* is more closely related antigenically to *E.sennetsu* than to *E. canis*. Further studies revealed no cross-reactivity between *E. risticii* and the granulocytic equine pathogen, *E. equi* [11, 25]. In addition, similar to

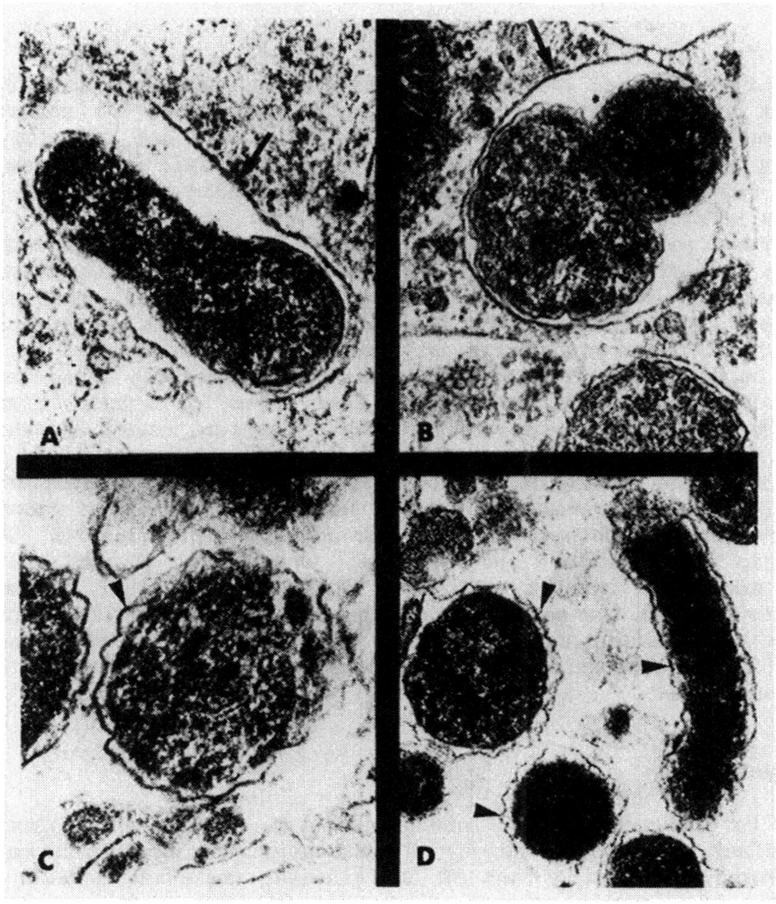

Figure 2. Electron micrograph of *Ehrlichia risticii* in P388D$_1$ cell cultures. Single microorganisms and inclusions are surrounded by a distinct cytoplasmic vacuolar membrane (A and B, arrows). Note the highly rippled outer membrane (C, D) and high degree of pleomorphism (D) of the microorganism.

other ehrlichiae, no cross-reactivity was demonstrated between *E. risticii* and 12 common *Rickettsia spp* [25]. Western blot analysis of *E. risticii* and *E. sennetsu* antigens revealed 11 common polypeptides. Four of these are considered to be dominant antigenic components. In a recent study conducted by Rikihisa *et al.* [22], two ponies were experimentally inoculated with live *E. sennetsu*. Although the infection proved asymptomatic, a strong humoral antibody response was elicited against both *E. sennetsu* and *E. risticii* as determined by the IFA test and Western immunoblot analysis. Subsequent challenge with live *E. risticii* resulted in the clinical protection of these ponies against EME, thereby providing evidence that at least some of the *E. sennetsu* antigens common to *E. risticii* are cross-protective.

A number of studies indicated that mice [23], dogs [26], cats [5], and nonhuman primates (rhesus monkeys) are susceptible to experimental infection with *E. risticii*. Of these, only mice and, possibly, cats show any clinical signs of disease [5, 33]. Field seroepidemiologic studies have indicated that foxes and wild rabbits may also be susceptible to infection with *E. risticii*.

The known geographic distribution of *E. risticii* and, consequently, EME, is rapidly increasing. Whether the disease has been newly introduced in various regions or simply misdiagnosed remains to be determined. Nevertheless, EME has now been diagnosed in 38 states of the United States, in bordering provinces of Canada, and in France [25]. In addition, seroepidemiologic studies currently being conducted provide strong evidence that EME is also affecting horses in southern Italy [Holland *et al.*, unpublished data]. The most recent states of the U.S. to be included are Arizona, Alaska, and Hawaii.

Thus far, the biological vector responsible for transmission of *E. risticii* in nature remains elusive. Based on information known about other ehrlichial agents (e.g., *E. canis* and *E. phagocytophila*) [24], the geographic distribution and seasonal occurrence of EME [26] and susceptible host species [1], the American dog tick, *Dermacentor varibilis*, seemed the most likely suspect. However, studies conducted to date have failed to incriminate this arthopod as the biological vector [28]. Nevertheless, an arthropod vector remains suspect and the search continues.

Pathophysiology

Similar to other ehrlichial infections (e.g., canine ehrlichiosis) EME may manifest itself by a variety of syndromes, ranging from asymptomatic to a severe fulminating form of the disease, including some or all of the clinical signs previously mentioned [8, 35]. One of the most unusual clinical signs with respect to rickettsial infections that is associated with EME is diarrhea, which may occur in approximately 40-45% of clinically affected horses [34]. This diarrhea may range from mild to profuse watery ("pipestream") in nature. Whereby EME is primarily a bloodborne infection, studies have shown that, after the early phase of infection, *E. risticii* may become targeted to various tissues and organs including, but not limited to, the wall of the large colon, small colon, cecum, ileum, and mesenteric and colonic lymph nodes [14, 20]. A peroxidase-labelled, anti-*E. risticii* serum was prepared for use on paraffin sections of intestine derived from *E. risticii*-infected horses. During the acute phase of EME, *E. risticii* was identified within the cytoplasm of crypt epithelial cells and macrophages within the lamina propria and submucosa primarily of the large colon and, to a lesser degree, within the small colon, cecum and small colon, cecum and small intestine. By electron microscopy, the microorganisms were found within these organs in mast cells as well as the above cell types. While little or no gross pathological alterations are observable upon necropsy of affected animals [14, 35], it appears that the diarrhea may be the result of an electrolyte imbalance created during localized infection of cells within the gastrointestinal tract. According to a follow-up study conducted by Rikihisa *et al.*[22], microscopic examination of sections of the large colon of infected horses revealed focal degeneration and/or dedifferentiation and hyperplasia of glandular epithelial cells, depletion of goblet and Paneth cells, and monocytic infiltration. This infection resulted in a net lack of Na^+ and Cl^- movement within the colon.

In addition to the above findings, recent studies have determined that *E. risticii* can also be transmitted transplacentally to the fetus of infected mares [3]. Precolostral *E. risticii*-specific antibodies were detected in some foals born to mares with a history of naturally acquired PHF at some point during gestation [4, 29]. Subsequently, *E. risticii* was isolated from the bone marrow, spleen, mesenteric, and colonic lymph nodes of a 7-month fetus whose dam was experimentally infected at 3 months of gestation [3, 4]. However, the microorganism was not isolated from the corresponding tissues of the dam.

In the past few years since the recognition of EME, veterinarians have noticed an increasing incidence of abortions in mares after clinical EME [29]. Necropsy results of aborted fetuses, along with routine uterine cultures and biopsies and various blood assays from affected mares to determine the etiology, have been inconclusive. One case concerned a thoroughbred broodmare in Kentucky [4]. This mare developed PHF at 2 months gestation and aborted a nearly full-term fetus at 10 3/4 months gestation. Gross pathologic examination of the fetus revealed partially aerated lungs, tracheal froth, and hemorrhage in the shoulder joint. The amnion showed infarcts and calcified plaques. No significant histopathologic changes or adventitious bacteria were observed or cultured by standard bacteriological techniques. A serum sample collected from the fetus was negative for equine rhinopneumonitis virus and various leptospira species, but strongly positive against *E. risticii* at a titer of 1:320. At the time of abortion, the dam was serologically positive at a titer of 1:2560 against *E. risticii*. Thus, transplacental infections of the fetus may occur when mares are exposed to *E. risticii* during gestation. The frequency, extent, and overall effects of such infections are currently being studied.

Various studies have determined that tetracycline, administered at a dosage of 3 mg/lb/day for 5 to 10 days, is effective in the treatment of horses with EME [18]. Other supportive therapy, such as fluids and electrolytes, should also be administered when indicated.

Immunity

Similar to other rickettsiae, immunity to *E. risticii* appears to depend primarily on the cell-mediated immune response (CMI) rather than on humoral immunity [2, 17, 30]. In various studies conducted on protective immunity to *E. risticii*, recovery from infection results in resistance to clinical disease after homologous challenge [2, 8, 35]. Further, similar to the immunity induced by infection with *E. equi* [17], protective immunity to *E. risticii* appears to be of the sterile type since all attempts to recover the microorganism from the blood and solid tissues (e.g., spleen, liver, bone marrow and colonic/mesenteric lymph nodes) have failed [26]. Based on this premise, a killed vaccine (PHF-

Vax; Schering Corporation) was commercially developed and has proven thus far to be highly effective in protecting against EME both experimentally [27] and under field conditions, provided annual booster doses are administered.

Conclusion

Over the past 5 years, much knowledge has been gained on the pathophysiology of EME. Methods for chemotherapy and immunoprophylaxis have led to a significant decrease in mortality rates and in the number of clinical cases of EME. However, much research on *E. risticii* is needed to identify the putative biological vector(s), to determine the geographical distribution, and to develop a suitable rapid and specific diagnostic test for use under field conditions. Additional studies of *in-utero* transmission and fetal infections will enhance our understanding of the pathogenic properties of the ehrlichiae.

Ehrlichia risticii, and the disease which it causes, has undoubtedly been around for many years awaiting discovery. Similarly, there are probably a number of other unique ehrlichial agents remaining to be recognized that will serve to underscore the biologic and medical importance of the genus *Ehrlichia*.

References

1. **Carrol, J. F., and E. T. Schmidtmann.** 1986. Summer activity of the American dog tick, *Dermacentor variabilis* say, on equine premises enzootic for Potomac horse fever in central Maryland. *J. Econ. Entomol.* **79:** 62-66.
2. **Clements, M. L., C. L. Wisseman, Jr., T. E. Woodward, P. Fiset, J. S. Dumler, W. McNamee, R. E. Black, J. Rooney, T. P. Hughes, and M. M. Levine.** 1983. Reactogenicity, immunogenicity and efficacy of a chick embryo cell-derived vaccine for Rocky Mountain spotted fever. *J. Infect. Dis.* **148:**922-930.
3. **Dawson, J. E., M. Ristic, C. J. Holland, R. H. Whitlock, and J. E. Sessions.** 1987. Isolation of *Ehrlichia risticii*, causative agent of Potomac horse fever, from the fetus of an experimentally infected mare. *Vet. Rec.* **121:**232.
4. **Dawson, J. E., M. Ristic, C. J. Holland, R. H. Whitlock, and J. E. Sessions.** 1988. Isolation of *Ehrlichia risticii* from the fetus of a mare with Potomac horse fever. *Proc. Fifth Int. Conf. Equine Inf. Dis.*, pp. 213-216. Lexington, Kentucky.
5. **Dawson, J. E., I. Abeygunawardena, C. J. Holland, M. Buese, M. Ristic.** 1988a. Susceptibility of cats to infection with *Ehrlichia risticii*, causative agent of equine monocytic ehrlichiosis. *Am. J. Vet. Res.* **49:**2096-2100.
6. **Dutta, S. K., A. C. Myrup, R. M. Rice, M. G. Robl, and R. C. Hammond.** 1985. Experimental reproduction of Potomac horse fever in horses with a newly isolated *Ehrlichia* organism. *J. Clin. Microbiol.* **22:**265-269.

7. **Ehrich, M., B. D. Perry, H. F. Troutt, R. W. Dellers, and R. A. Magnusson.** 1984. Acute diarrhea in horses of the Potomac River area: examination for clostridial toxins. *J. Am. Vet. Med. Assoc.* **185**:433-435.
8. **Goetz, T. E., C. J. Holland, M. Ristic, K. Skibbe, K. Keegan, P. Johnson, D. Schaeffer, and G. Baker.** 1989. Prevalence and seasonal trend of indirect fluorescent antibody titers of apparently healthy Illinois horses against equine monocytic ehrlichiosis (synonym - Potomac horse fever) in 1986. *Am. J. Vet. Res.* In Press.
9. **Holland, C. J., M. Ristic, A. I. Cole, P. Johnson, G. Baker, and T. Goetz.** 1985. Isolation, experimental transmission, and characterization of causative agent of Potomac horse fever. *Science* **227**:522-524.
10. **Holland, C. J., M. Ristic, D. L. Huxsoll, A. I. Cole, and G. Rapmund.** 1985a. Adaptation of *Ehrlichia sennetsu* to canine blood monocytes: preliminary structural and serologic studies with cell culture-derived *Ehrlichia sennetsu*. *Infect. Immun.* **48**:366-371.
11. **Holland, C. J., E. Weiss, W. Burgdorfer, A. I. Cole, and I. Kakoma.** 1985b. *Ehrlichia risticii* sp. nov.: etiologic agent of equine monocytic ehrlichiosis (synonym, Potomac horse fever). *Int. J. Syst. Bacteriol.* **35**:524-526.
12. **Huang, J. C. M., S. L. Wright, and W. D. Shipley.** 1983. Isolation of a corona virus-like agent from horses suffering from acute equine diarrhoea. *Vet. Rec.* **113**:262-263.
13. **Jenny, A. L.** 1984. Potomac horse fever - National Veterinary Services Laboratories (USDA) Report. *Amer. Assoc. Equine Practnr. Newsltr* **No.2**:64-66.
14. **Johnson, G. C., and Y. Rikihisa.** 1988. Intestinal pathology of murine *Ehrlichia risticii* infection. *Abst. Proc. Third Equine Res. Colic Symp.* Athens, GA.
15. **Knowles, R. C., D. W. Anderson, W. D. Shipley, R. H. Whitlock, B. D. Perry, and J. P. Davidson.** 1983. Acute equine diarrhea syndrome (AEDS): a preliminary report. *Proc. Am. Assoc. Equine Pract.* **29**:353-357.
16. **Nyindo, M. B. A., M. Ristic, D. L. Huxsoll, and A. R. Smith.** 1971. Tropical canine pancytopenia: *in-vitro* cultivation of the causative agent - *Ehrlichia canis*. *Am. J. Vet. Res.* **32**:1651-1658.
17. **Nyindo, M. B. A., M. Ristic, G. E. Lewis, Jr., D. L. Huxsoll, and E. H. Stephenson.** 1978. Immune responses of ponies to experimental infection with *Ehrlichia equi*. *Am. J. Vet. Med. Res.* **39**:15-18.
18. **Palmer, J. E., R. H. Whitlock, and C. E. Benson.** 1988. Clinical signs and treatment of equine ehrlichial colitis. *Proc. Symp. on Potomac horse fever*, pp. 49-54. Louisville, Kentucky.
19. **Rikihisa, Y., and B. D. Perry.** 1985. Causative ehrlichial organisms in Potomac horse fever. *Infect. Immun.* **49**:513-517.
20. **Rikihisa, Y., B. D. Perry, and D. O. Cordes.** 1985a. Ultrastructural study of ehrlichial organisms in the large colons of ponies infected with Potomac horse fever. *Infect. Immun.* **49**:505-512.
21. **Rikihisa, Y., and B. M. Jiang.** 1988. *In-vitro* susceptibility of

*Ehrlichia ristici*i to eight antibiotics. *Antimicrob. Agents Chemother.* **32**:986-991.

22. **Rikihisa, Y., C. I. Pretzman, G. C. Johnson, S. M. Reed, S. Y. Yamamoto, and F. Andrews.** 1988. Clinical, histopathological, and immunological responses of ponies to *Ehrlichia sennetsu* and subsequent *Ehrlichia risticii* challenge. *Infect. Immun.* **56**:2960-2966.
23. **Rikihisa, Y., G. Johnson, H. J. Cook, and S. M. Reed.** 1988a. Pathophysiologic changes of large colon of horses infected with *Ehrlichia risticii*. *Abst. Proc. Third Equine Res. Colic. Symp.* Athens, GA.
24. **Ristic, M., and D. L. Huxsoll.** 1984. *Ehrlichieae*, pp. 704-709 *In* Bergey's Manual of Systematic Bacteriology, Vol. 1., N. R. Krieg and J. G. Holt (eds). The Williams and Wilkens Co., Baltimore, MD.
25. **Ristic, M., C. J. Holland, J. E. Dawson, J. Sessions, and J. E. Palmer.** 1986. Diagnosis of equine monocytic ehrlichiosis (syn. Potomac horse fever) by indirect immunofluorescence. *J. Am. Vet. Med. Assoc.* **189**:39-46.
26. **Ristic, M., J. E. Dawson, C. J. Holland, A. L. Jenny.** 1988. Susceptibility of dogs to infection with *Ehrlichia risticii*, causative agent of equine monocytic ehrlichiosis (Potomac horse fever). *Am. J. Vet. Res.* **49**:1497-1500.
27. **Ristic, M., C. J. Holland, and T. E. Goetz.** 1988a. Evaluation of a vaccine for equine monocytic ehrlichiosis. *Proc. Vth Int. Conf. on Equine Infect. Dis.*, pp. 206-213. University Press, Lexington, KY.
28. **Schmidtmann, E. T., M. G. Robl, J. F. Carroll.** 1986. Attempted transmission of *Ehrlichia risticii* by field-captured *Dermacentor variabilis (Acari:Ixodidae)*. *Am. J. Vet. Res.* **47**:2393-2395.
29. **Sessions, J. E.** 1988. Potomac horse fever field studies in Maryland and on an endemic farm. *Proc. Symp. on Potomac horse fever*, pp. 79-87. Louisville, Kentucky.
30. **Shirai, A., V. Sankakran, E. Gan, and D. L. Huxsoll.** 1978. Early detection of *Rickettsia tsutsugamushi* in peripheral monocyte cultures derived from experimentally infected monkeys and dogs. *Southeast Asian J. Trop. Med. Pub. Health.* **9**:11-14.
31. **Weiss, E., G. A. Dasch, U. H. Kang, and H. N. Westfall.** 1985. Biological properties of host cell-free *Ehrlichia sennetsu*. *Abst. Workshop on Diseases Caused by Leukocytic Rickettsiae of Man and Animals*, pp. 18. Urbana, IL.
32. **Weiss, E., G. A. Dasch, Y. H. Kang, and H. N. Westfall.** 1988. Substrate utilization by *Ehrlichia sennetsu* and *Ehrlichia risticii* separated from host constituents by renografin gradient centrifugation. *J. Bacteriol.* **170**:5012-5017.
33. **Wells, M. Y., and Y. Rikihisa.** 1988. Lack of lysosomal fusion with phagosomes containing *Ehrlichia risticii* in P388D1 cells: Abrogation of inhibition with tetracycline. *Infect. Immun.* **56**:3209-3215.
34. **Whitlock, R. H., J. E. Palmer, C. E. Benson, H. M. Acland, A. L. Jenny, and M. Ristic.** 1984. Potomac horse fever: clinical characteristics and diagnostic features. *Am. Assoc. Vet. Lab. Diagnosticians, 27th Annu. Proceedings,* pp. 103-124.

35. **Whitlock, R. H., B. Perry, A. Jenny, J. E. Palmer, M. Ristic, E. T. Schmidtmann, C. J. Holland, J. E. Sessions, M. Robl, Y. Rikihisa, C. Benson, S. K. Dutta, and R. Meinersmann.** 1985. Potomac horse fever: update and research priorities. *Proc. 89th Annu. Mtg. U.S. Anim. Health Assoc.*, pp. 23-29. Milwaukee, WI.

7. PATHOPHYSIOLOGY OF CANINE EHRLICHIOSIS

Indira Abeygunawardena, D.V.M., M.S.
I. Kakoma, D.V.M., Ph.D.
R. D. Smith, D.V.M., Ph.D.

Abstract

The pathogenesis of canine ehrlichiosis or tropical canine pancytopenia (TCP) involves a wide range of effector mechanisms targeted to mature platelets and thrombocytes. The predominant mechanisms are immunologically mediated resulting in platelet sequestration coincident with significant reduction in the number of circulating platelets. Another pathway involving the platelet migration inhibition factor (PMIF) has been identified to play a key role in the pathogenesis of TCP by enhancing platelet sequestration and stasis, leading to reduced peripheral platelet count and probably hemorrhagic diatheses. PMIF is associated with virulence and partially characterized as a thermostable glycoprotein elevated in body fluids of dogs severely affected by mild strains of *Ehrlichia canis*.

Introduction

Canine ehrlichiosis, or tropical canine pancytopenia (TCP), is a tick-borne disease of the canidae. TCP presents with a variety of individual and breed-related clinical manifestations ranging from mild to acute and chronic forms of the disease (see Chapter 1, Fig. 2). Typically, there is a pancytopenia mainly affecting the platelets (Fig. 1). In adult dogs, the mild form is common, whereas puppies suffer a severe disease [5]. Buhles *et al.* [2] categorized the syndrome into different phases. The acute phase occurs in both Beagle and German sheperd dogs during the first 2 to 4 weeks and is characterized by mild signs and transient pancytopenia. Beagle dogs are considerably more resistance to the disease which progresses into a mild chronic state. German shepherd dogs are highly susceptible and tend to have severe pancytopenia, hemorrhage (e.g., epistaxis), and peripheral edema due to a prolonged course of infection and pathogenetic responses. The latter form of the disease has been termed severe chronic and is often fatal due to excessive bleeding [11]. In general, mixed breed and beagle dogs are less susceptible to the severe chronic form of the disease [11].

Pathogenesis of the pancytopenia has received extensive attention but remains poorly defined. Burghen *et al.* [3] suggested that platelet destruction is related to immunological processes. The characteristic hypergammaglobulinemia [2, 3], systemic plasmacytosis, and observation that specific antibody does not correlate with protection led Weisiger *et al.* [21] to suggest that the immune response may enhance the pathogenesis of ehrlichiosis [3]. These authors suggested that the

J. C. Williams and I. Kakoma (eds.), Ehrlichiosis, 78–92.

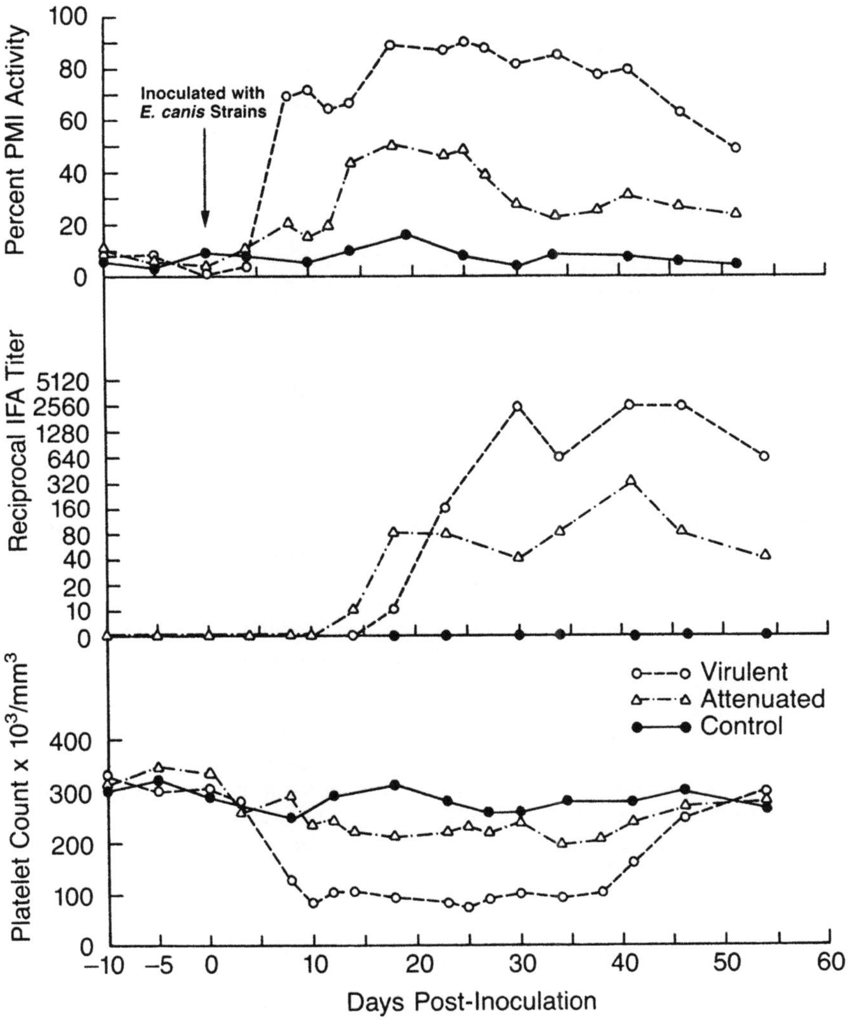

Figure 1. Temporal relationship between platelet count, IFA titers, and PMI activity.

hypergammaglobulinemia may be related to a state of autoimmunity induced by the infection. This hypothesis has been supported by Hildebrandt *et al.* [9] and Ristic *et al.* [16]. The role of anti-ehrlichia antibody may be in the pathogenesis of the disease, suggesting that a blocking antibody protected the microorganism from destruction by the immune system.

Thrombokinetic studies by Smith *et al.* [17, 18, 19, 20], Smith and Kakoma [17], and radioisotope studies on the bone marrow by Buhles *et al.* [2] have implicated depression or malfunction of the bone marrow precursor cells as the primary disorder leading to thrombocytopenia.

Many of these studies suggest that thrombocytopenia may be the result of decreased platelet life span, possibly related to the immune response, involving direct and indirect effects of autoimmunity on a wide range of target cells, particularly the thrombocytes [12, 13].

Experimental Basis

The major experiments have investigated the roles of hypersplenism, reduced thrombopoiesis, and increased platelet destruction under the hypothesis that "thrombocytopenia is the result of or a combination effect of splenic pooling, reduced platelet production and accelerated platelet destruction."

In all cases, every effort was made to save the animals according to recommendations for humane use of experimental animals.

Hypersplenism

The circulating platelet compartment is in equilibrium with an exchangeable splenic pool [6, 7, 8]. Hypersplenism, leading to increased pooling of platelets in an oversized spleen, has been suggested as a cause of thrombocytopenia on the basis of the finding of splenomegaly in *E. canis*-infected dogs. In humans, hypersplenism has been associated with cirrhosis, congestive splenomegaly, myelofibrosis, chronic lymphatic leukemia, Hodgkin's disease, and lymphosarcoma. Radiolabeled platelet survival may be normal or only slightly reduced, but body surface scanning reveals a pronounced increase in spleen surface radioactivity. Thus the thrombocytopenia associated with splenomegaly is primarily due to maldistribution rather than diminished production or accelerated destruction of platelets. The primary site of ^{51}Cr-labeled platelet destruction in *E. canis*-infected dogs is the spleen [19, 20]. Splenectomy results in an increase in circulating platelet counts.

Decreased Platelet Production

Decreased platelet production may result from megakaryocyte hypoproliferation, i.e., marrow hypoplasia or replacement, or decreased platelet production per nuclear unit, i.e., ineffective thrombopoiesis [6, 7, 8]. Marrow hypoplasia has been reported in *E. canis*-infected dogs on the basis of necropsy findings [9] and persistence of pancytopenia after therapeutic removal of the agent from chronically infected dogs [2]. In humans, megakaryocyte aplasia or hypoplasia can be induced by drug, radiation, infections, genetic, or idiopathic damage to the marrow [6, 7]. Infectious diseases include bacterial endocarditis, malaria, leptospirosis, tuberculosis, acute hepatitis, and bacterial septicemias. Most infections inducing thrombocytopenia by marrow hypoplasia are also accompanied by increased platelet destruction [6, 7, 8].

Increased Platelet Destruction

Radiolabeled platelet survival data have clearly shown that platelets are removed at an accelerated rate in *E. canis*-infected dogs [18, 19, 20]. Accelerated platelet removal may result from platelet consumption associated with inflammatory changes in blood vessel endothelium or through disseminated intravascular coagulation. Other studies have suggested direct immunologically mediated destruction of platelets [12, 13].

Relationship with Various Human Thrombocytopathies

Tropical canine pancytopenia is potentially a useful model for human idiopathic thrombocytopenia and autoimmune mechanisms of putatively similar etiology. In Table 1, a modification from Harker [6, 7, 8], typical platelet profiles are shown, and Table 2 shows comparable data in TCP-afflicted dogs. As discussed by Smith and Kakoma [17], these results have striking similarities and should be seriously explored as a model for human and other animal diseases with an autoimmune component.

TABLE 1. Typical platelet profiles in various human thrombocytopathies.

Condition	Count	Survival (days)	Turnover (x normal)
Normal	250,000	9.50	1.0
Splenic pooling	75,000	8.00	2.0
Hypoproliferation	25,000	7.00	0.1
Ineffective thrombopoiesis	50,000	9.00	0.2
Immune destruction	10,000	0.05	7.0
Consumption	25,000	0.20	4.0

Typically, a portion of ^{51}Cr-labeled platelets, equivalent to the size of the splenic pool, is lost from the circulation within a few hours of transfusion [6]. A much higher percentage of labeled platelets was recovered from uninfected dogs (76.9%) than from *E. canis*-infected dogs (39.4%), equivalent to 23.1 and 60.6% pooling, respectively. Estimates

TABLE 2. Platelet kinetics in three normal and three *E. canis*-infected dogs.

Dog	Platelet count/ml	Platelet survival (days)	Platelet recovery %	Turnover (platelets/ml per day)	Effective production (x normal)
Normal	277,000	6.76	76.9	49,122	1.000
Infected	48,667	1.36	39.4	80,378	1.633

of the degree of splenic pooling after splenectomy of normal and *E. canis*-infected dogs (24 and 62%, respectively) closely approximate those derived from ^{51}Cr-labeled platelet survival studies. Thus, there is good evidence that increased splenic pooling, or hypersplenism, contributes to thrombocytopenia in canine ehrlichiosis. However, splenectomy does not appear to significantly affect the course of canine ehrlichiosis.

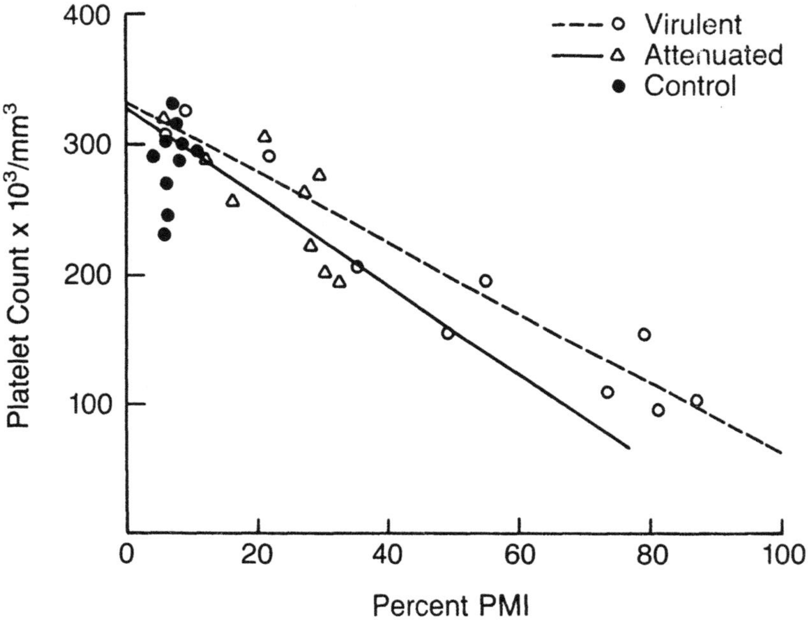

Figure 2. Correlation between platelet count and PMI response in dogs inoculated with virulent, compared with control (normal) dogs.

Simulation Studies on Platelet Kinetics in TCP

Description of the model

Platelet production and destruction were simulated by an age-class model (available upon request) consisting of two marrow compartments and eight circulating platelet compartments. The marrow compartments simulated the reported 2-day delay between a stimulus and an increase in the number of platelets released from the marrow [6, 7, 8]. Circulating platelets are removed by a random process, representing consumption, before movement to the next compartment. The rate of random removal was estimated empirically by the best fit of simulation data to actual ^{51}Cr-labeled platelet survival data in normal and experimentally infected dogs. After passing through all eight circulating platelet compartments, platelets are assumed to die as a result of senescence.

Platelets are assumed to move freely between the circulating and splenic compartments, with approximately 77% of platelets in the general circulation and 23% in the splenic pool at any given instant (Table 2). The size of the splenic pool in *E. canis*-infected dogs was estimated to be approximately 61%. Homeostatic mechanisms are assumed to be responsive to the total platelet mass, circulating and splenic [6]. Forces responsible for random removal of platelets are considered to act upon both compartments, and all age groups are considered to be equally affected.

Simulations

Simulation experiments were performed in a sequence whereby estimates of variables derived in one step were incorporated into the next. The resulting data were compared visually with experimental data, and the degree of agreement, or validity, was determined by linear regression analysis [6, 7, 8]. Values for parameters providing the best fit to experimental data are summarized below.

Platelet survival

Typically, there is a pancytopenia mainly affecting the platelets (Fig. 1). A random rate of platelet removal of -0.2614 (equivalent to removal of 23% of the platelet mass per day) provided a very close fit of simulated to actual ^{51}Cr-labeled platelet survival data for three normal dogs, with a coefficient of correlation (r^2) of 0.98 (Fig. 2). The corresponding value for three infected dogs was -0.7133 (equivalent to removal of 51% of the platelet mass per day), with a coefficient of determination of 0.99.

Splenic pooling

The simulated postsplenectomy platelet count for four normal dogs was 415,178/ml, 1.4% less than the observed count of 421,000/ml. The simulated platelet count for five *E. canis*-infected dogs was 160,875/ml, which was 4.5% less than the observed value of 168,500/ml. The finding that postsplenectomy platelet counts of normal and *E. canis*-infected dogs were within 5% of expected values confirms that the initial loss of ^{51}Cr-labeled platelets is due entirely to sequestration in an exchangeable splenic pool. The size of this pool increases after infection.

Simulation of the rate of onset and severity of thrombocytopenia in E. canis-infected dogs

The simulated platelet count stabilized at 53,085/ml 14 days postinfection, 10.9% below the value of 59,571/ml measured in 12 experimentally infected dogs. Holding platelet turnover unchanged at 140,700/ml per day before and after simulated infection provided the best fit to actual data. The difference in the rate of onset of thrombocytopenia between simulated and actual data was not surprising, as pathologic mechanisms invoked by *E. canis* probably develop gradually, versus the abrupt change inherent in the model. Although a gradual onset of thrombocytopenia could be simulated, it would not alter the validity of the conclusions.

The Contribution of Simulation Studies

As detailed by Smith and Kakoma [17], simulation studies demonstrated that (a) on the average, there was a 2.7 factor increase in platelet removal and sequestration in *E. canis*-infected dogs above normal ranges. This was statistically correlated with the genesis and magnitude of thrombocytopenia; (b) apparently the effects on thrombopoiesis and function were operative at the bone marrow level. These characteristics are summarized in Tables 1 and 2.

In-Vitro and In-Vivo Studies

The platelet migration inhibition test (PMIT) has been used qualitatively and quantitatively to compare the relative virulence of defined strains of *E. canis* in highly susceptible dogs [1]. These experiments involved purification of the PMIF and determining the type of leukocyte that synthesized and released the factor. In addition, the relationship between specific antibody response and PMIF were investigated.

Platelet Migration Inhibition Test (PMIT)

A modification of the technique of Dequesnoy *et al.* [4] was used. About 20 ml of blood was drawn from a normal dog into 2 ml of 20% sodium citrate in 0.15 M NaC1. The blood was centrifuged at 500 x g for 20 min at room temperature. The upper two-thirds of the platelet-rich plasma (PRP) layer was removed and centrifuged at 1,200 x g for 20 min to prepare platelet-poor plasma (PPP) and the platelet pellet. The platelet pellet was resuspended in 1 ml of PPP. The remaining PPP was saved for the PMIT.

A 200 ml platelet suspension containing 1 to 2 x 10^8 platelets/ml was mixed with 300 ml heat-inactivated test serum. After incubation at room temperature for 60 min, the mixture was placed in a glass microcapillary tube (2 ml). One end of the tube was heat-sealed and centrifuged at 700 x g for 3 min. The tubes were cut approximately 1 mm above the surface of the platelet button. The stumps containing platelets were anchored with silicon grease in the center of a 25-m coverslip which served as the floor of the migration chambers. The migration chambers were covered with a second coverslip and filled with medium containing 300 ml of minimum essential medium (MEM), 200 ml of autologous PPP (heat-inactivated at 56°C for 30 min and clarified by centrifugation at 750 x g for 30 min to remove debris), and supplemented with 100 units of penicillin and 10 mg of streptomycin. The chambers were incubated at 37°C for 18 hours, and areas of migration were measured by a light microscope equipped with a calibrated ocular micrometer at 40X magnification. The mean percent migration inhibition for each postinoculation serum sample, relative to the migration area of platelets incubated with preinoculation sera, was calculated by the following formula:

$$\text{PMI (I)} = 100 - \frac{D1}{D2} \times 100$$

Where D1 = mean diameter of platelet migration in presence of postinoculation (test) serum; and D_2 = mean diameter of platelet migration in presence of preinoculation (normal) serum. All tests were done in triplicate and results were based on the mean of three observations for each serum sample.

Indirect Immunofluorescent Antibody (IFA) Test

The test was performed on all sera by the standard method [14, 15, 16, 21].

Production of PMIF by Lymphocyte Co-culture with Infected Monocytes

Infected monocytes and lymphocyte cultures were prepared from a male pointer proven to be free from ehrlichiosis. Uninfected monocyte and lymphocyte cultures were prepared from another normal *E. canis*-free dog.

Preparation of Lymphocyte Cultures

Lymphocytes were separated from peripheral blood by the Ficoll Hypaque gradient method of Ho and Babiuk [10]. The interface containing lymphocytes was washed with Hanks balanced salt solution (HBSS) and resuspended in M199 medium containing 20% heat-inactivated canine serum. The cell suspension was incubated in tissue culture flasks in a humidified CO_2 incubator to remove contaminating adherent cells. The nonadherent cell suspension, operationally referred to as lymphocytes, was maintained in cultures. Culture supernatant fluids were harvested every 2 days and tested for PMIF.

Preparation of Monocyte Cultures

Infected and uninfected monocytes were cultured as described by Nyindo *et al.* [14]. Briefly, blood was collected into a dextran-heparin mixture. After red blood cell sedimentation, leukocyte-rich plasma was placed in flasks. Nonadherent cells were discarded and adherent monocytes were supplemented with medium containing M199 medium, 1% L-glutamine, and 20% heat-inactivated canine serum. Similarly, the supernatant fluids were collected every 2 days and tested for PMIF.

Lymphocytes and monocytes were maintained individually as primary cultures as well. In addition, co-cultures of the two cell types were set up in different combinations to test for synergistic or inhibitory interaction of these cells in the induction of PMIF synthesis and release.

Partial Purification of PMIF from Sera of *E. canis*-Infected Dogs

For the preliminary purification, sera from infected dogs were fractionated on Sephadex G-200 (Pharmacia Fine Chemicals, Uppsala, Sweden). The elution profile was monitored at 280 nm and fractions constituting a single peak were pooled and concentrated to the starting sample volume. Each of the resultant three peaks were tested for PMI activity. Normal canine serum was similarly fractionated and tested for comparative purposes.

The second peak from Sephadex G-200 filtration, which was later shown to be positive for PMI activity, was further fractionated by immunoaffinity chromatography with Protein A conjugated to cyanogen bromide-activated Sepharose CL-4B (Pharmacia Fine Chemicals, Uppsala, Sweden). The first peak, which was devoid of IgG, was eluted with 0.1 M $NaHCO_3$, pH 8.0. IgG bound to Protein A was eluted with 10 ml of 0.2 M Na_2CO_3, pH 11.5. The optical density at 280 nm was determined for each fraction and those appearing to constitute a single peak were pooled and concentrated. Both peaks were tested for PMI activity and IFA reactivity.

Results and Relevance of In-Vivo and In-Vitro Studies to the Pathogenesis of Canine Ehrlichiosis

Dogs inoculated with the virulent strain showed mild fever, depression, and anorexia. Moreover, they showed a dramatic and significant decrease ($p < 0.015$) in platelet numbers, which usually fell below 100,000/ml by 15 to 20 days after inoculation and persisted for 20 to 25 days at low levels. None of the dogs inoculated with the attenuated *E. canis* strain showed evidence of clinical disease. Figure 1 shows the temporal relationship between IFA, PMI, and platelet count.

Animals in both treatment groups were positive in the PMIT 7 days after inoculation. Analysis of variance of PMIT data from the study showed a significant ($p < 0.05$) increase in inhibition of platelet migration above baseline values (6.2%) in dogs inoculated with the virulent agent. Their PMI response continued to rise for 2 weeks to a maximum of approximately 90%, whereas dogs that received the attenuated agent exhibited a maximum inhibitory effect of 37% by Day 15. Anti-*E. canis* antibody titers became evident about 4 to 5 days after initial PMI responses. The dogs that were inoculated with the virulent agent remained serologically positive at higher levels (1:2560) as compared with those inoculated with the attenuated agent. In addition, the former group kept the high IFA titers well after 55 days. Both control dogs remained seronegative throughout the experimental period.

By using regression analysis, significant negative correlations ($r = -0.96$ and $r = -0.70$ for virulent and attenuated agents, respectively) were found between platelet numbers and the percent of PMI (Fig. 2). Dogs inoculated with uninfected, transformed murine monocytes, and

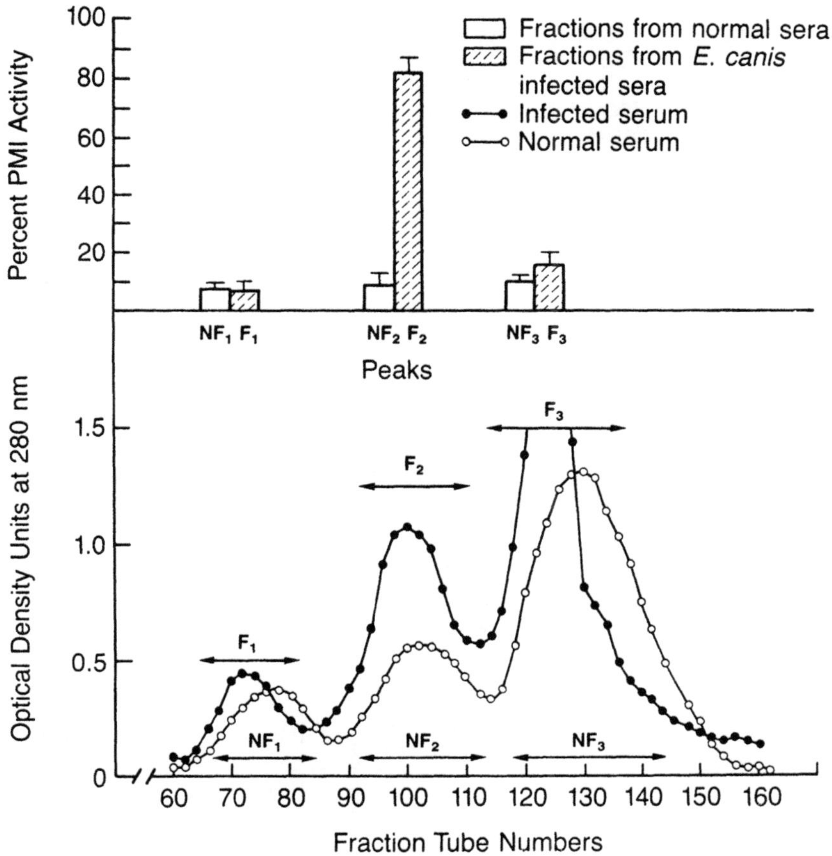

Figure 3. Elution profile of *E. canis*-infected serum and normal serum on Sephadex G-200. Highest PMI activity was observed in the peak (F_2) which co-eluted with IgG from sera of an *E. canis*-infected dog (mean % ± SE).

uninfected whole blood maintained normal platelet counts and baseline PMI values.

The PMIF activity was observed 5 to 6 days after initiating cultures. After 11 to 12 days, the cells started to degenerate and gradually lost PMI-producing ability.

Three protein peaks were obtained after fractionating sera from *E. canis*-infected dogs on Sephadex G-200. When the three peaks were assayed for PMIF, fraction F_2 showed the highest activity (Fig. 3). The degree of inhibition was four times higher than either of the other two peaks from the same sera. The three fractions of serum obtained from the control dog had negligible PMI activity (7.2% to 10.3%).

The second fraction from Sephadex G-200, with the highest PMI activity, was further purified by immunoaffinity chromatography on a Protein A column (Fig. 6). The first peak showed much higher inhibitory

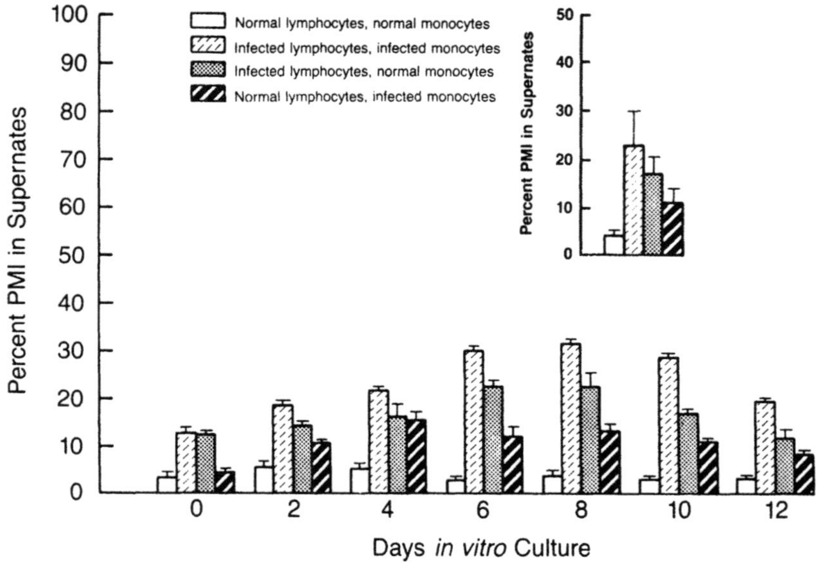

Figure 4. Influence of infected canine monocytes on the production of PMIF by normal canine lymphocytes (mean % ± SE). Inset: mean values over entire culture period.

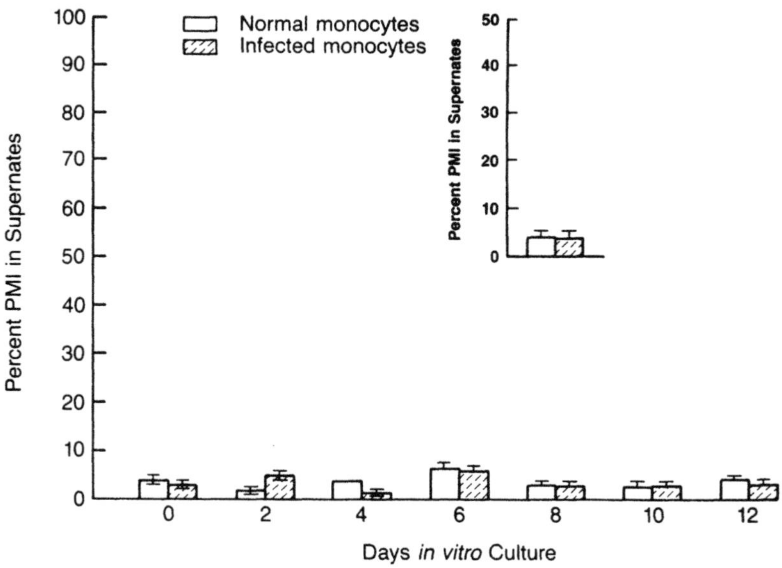

Figure 5. PMI activity of supernates derived from monocyte cultures prepared from an *E. canis*-infected dog and a normal dog (mean % ± SE). Inset: mean values over entire culture period. Note that no significant amount of PMIF was measured.

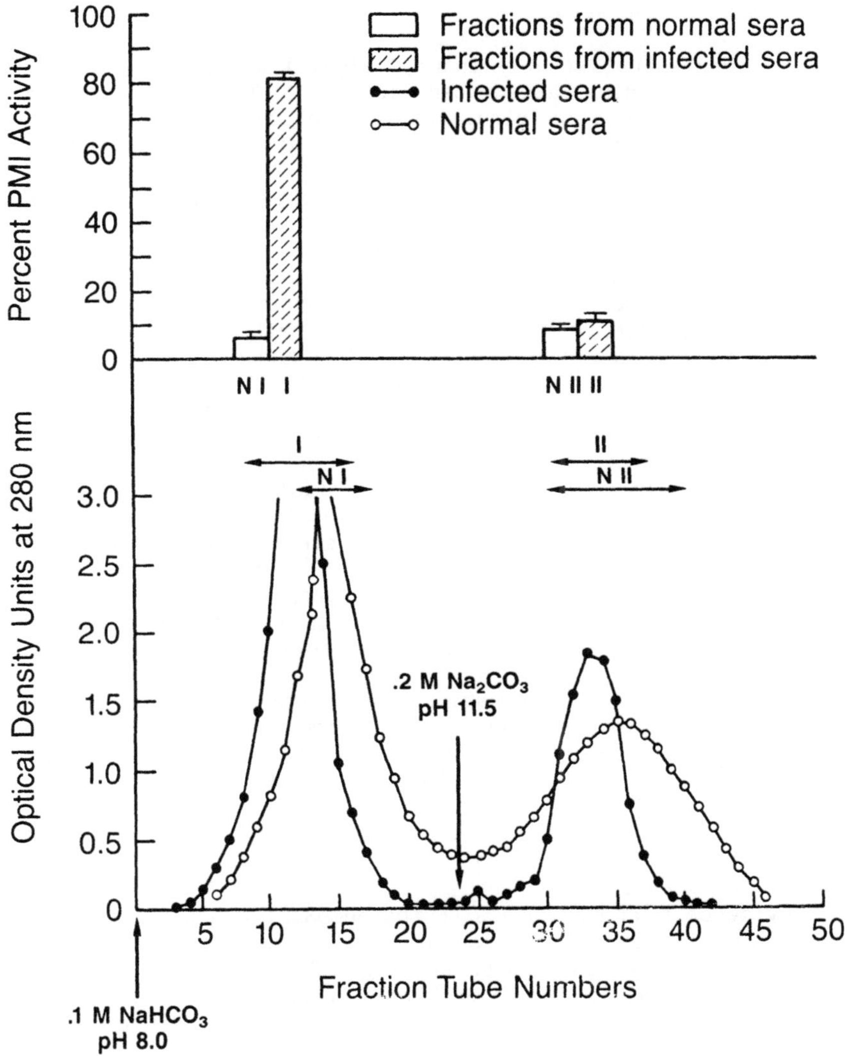

Figure 6. Elution profile from immunoaffinity chromatography of peak F from Sephadex G-200 column. Second peak which eluted at a high pH failed to induce PMIF response. However, it had antibody activity to *E. canis* (mean % ± SE).

activity. The PMI activity was demonstrated in an IgG-devoid peak lacking IFA reactivity against *E. canis* antigen.

We demonstrated that the synthesis of PMIF was largely attributable to lymphocyte function (Fig. 4) and that monocytes alone did not produce any significant amount of PMIF (Fig. 5).

Levels of PMIF in the serum

Virulent *E. canis* consistently induced significantly higher PMIF levels than the corresponding attenuated strain. The difference may be attributed to the loss of virulence of the latter isolate during its prolonged *in-vitro* propagation and passage in a murine monocyte cell line.

Although a characteristic humoral response pattern has been reported in dogs infected with *E. canis*, it does not seem to be associated with protective immunity [16, 21]. The same pattern seems to apply to the PMIF profile. However, the appearance of the latter factor precedes specific humoral responses and is more pronounced in severely infected dogs, indicating that PMIF is important in pathogenesis. This factor induces prominent surface changes [13] associated with platelet destruction contributing to thrombocytopenia in canine ehrlichiosis [12]. These results provide evidence that the quantity of PMIF is directly related to the magnitude of platelet destruction and virulence of a strain. Accordingly, PMIF might be useful as a prognostic indicator of the severity of canine ehrlichiosis.

Recent data have confirmed that, during *in-vitro* cultivation, lymphocytes, from *E. canis*-infected dogs, elaborate and release PMIF into the medium. Thus, it seems that PMIF is produced by activated lymphocytes. In addition, it seems reasonable to speculate that the immune stimulation of normal lymphocytes by infected monocytes may be mediated by either *E. canis*, its residual antigens, and/or unidentified mediators.

In an attempt to answer questions regarding the nature and role of PMIF *in vivo*, we have fractionated sera from infected dogs in order to isolate the active factor. In Sephadex G-200 chromatography, PMIF co-elutes with IgG at an estimated molecular weight range of 150 to 190.

The PMIF activity of a fraction isolated by immunoaffinity chromatography confirms that it is a non-IgG moiety as reported previously [12, 13], and its function is distinct from specific antibodies to *E. canis*.

Since evidence thus far points to the hemostatic and pathogenetic role of PMIF, knowledge on the antigenicity and immunogenicity of the factor would contribute to the understanding of the pathogenesis of the disease, and possibly to the immunoprophylactic and therapeutic potential of this intriguing molecule or groups of molecules.

Conclusion

Thrombocytopenia is consistently reported in dogs with ehrlichiosis and is a useful parameter for the diagnosis of the disease [23]. The rate and pattern of development of this hematological abnormality of infected dogs in *in-vivo* and *in-vitro* studies are consistent with previous findings [12, 13, 17-20]. Thrombocytopenia was evident in the experimental group inoculated with the virulent strain of the microorganism. It is noteworthy that dogs inoculated with attenuated microorganisms experienced relatively less of a decline in platelet counts.

Platelets are generally considered relatively mobile elements in the blood, drifting in the circulation until direct contact with damaged endothelial cells causes them to participate in hemostasis [6, 7, 8]. Based on platelet migration patterns demonstrated *in vitro*, it would be reasonable to speculate that this phenomenon has some physiological significance *in vivo* in the hemostatic process. This active migration of normal platelets appears to be inhibited by some soluble serum factor(s) associated with *E. canis* infection but is not found in uninfected normal canine sera [12, 13]. The factor has been designated as platelet migration inhibition factor (PMIF) [12] similar to that associated with human autoimmune disease [4]. The inhibitory factor has been shown by scanning electron microscopy to induce prominent platelet surface changes leading to increased vulnerability to direct destruction by the reticuloendothelial system [12, 13, 22, 23]. Thus, although PMIF may directly reduce normal involvement of platelets in hemostatic processes, the factor also induces surface changes which may accelerate platelet removal from the circulation.

As shown previously in our laboratories and reaffirmed in more recent *in-vivo* and *in-vitro* studies, nearly all *E. canis*-infected dogs have significantly ($p < 0.05$) increased levels of PMIF.

References

1. **Abeygunawardena, I.** 1987. Kinetics of the platelet migration inhibition factor in canine ehrlichiosis. *M.S. Thesis*, University of Illinois at Urbana-Champaign, IL.
2. **Buhles, W. C., D. L. Huxsoll, and P. K. Hildebrandt.** 1974. Tropical canine pancytopenia: clinical, hematologic, and serologic response of dogs to *Ehrlichia canis* infection, tetracycline therapy and challenge inoculation. *J. Infect. Dis.* **130**:357-367.
3. **Burghen, G. A., W. R. Beisel, J. S. Walker, R. M. Nims, D. L. Huxsoll, and P. K. Hildebrandt.** 1971. Development of hypergammaglobulinemia in tropical canine pancytopenia. *Am. J. Vet. Res.* **32**:749-756.
4. **Duquesnoy, R. J., D. F. Lorentzen, and R. H. Aster.** 1975. Platelet migration inhibition: a new method for detection of platelet antibodies. *Blood* **45**:741-747.
5. **Ewing, S. A.** Canine ehrlichiosis. 1969. Advances in Veterinary Medicine and Comparative Medicine, Vol. 13, pp. 331-353, C. A. Brandly and C. A. Cornelius, (eds.), Academic Press, Inc., NY.
6. **Harker, L. A.** 1970a. Platelet kinetics in man, pp. 174-184, *In* Formation and destruction of blood cells, T. J. Greenwalt and G. A. Jamieson (Eds.), J. B. Lippincott, Philadelphia, PA.
7. **Harker, L. A.** 1970b. Thrombokinetics in idiopathic thrombocytopenic purpura. *Br. J. Haematol.* **19**:95-104.
8. **Harker, L. A.** 1971. Platelet production and its regulation, pp. 202-211, *In* Platelet kinetics, J. M. Paulus (ed.), Elsevier, New York, NY.
9. **Hildebrandt, P. K., D. L. Huxsoll, J. S. Walker, R. M. Nims, R. Taylor, and M. Andrews.** 1973. Pathology of canine ehrlichiosis (tropical canine pancytopenia). *Am. J. Vet. Res.* **34**:1309-1320.

10. **Ho, C. K., and L. A. Babiuk.** 1978. Isolation of various canine leukocytes and their characterization by surface marker analysis. *Immunology* **35**:733-740.
11. **Huxsoll, D. L., H. L. Amyx, I. E. Hemelt, P. K. Hildebrandt, R. M. Nims, and W. S. Gochenour.** 1972. Laboratory studies of tropical canine pancytopenia. *Exp. Parasitol.* **31**:53-59.
12. **Kakoma, I., C. A. Carson, and M. Ristic.** 1980. Direct and indirect lymphocyte participation in the immunity and immunopathology of tropical canine pancytopenia--a review. *Comp. Immun. Microbiol. Infect. Dis.* **3**:291-298.
13. **Kakoma, I., C. A. Carson, M. Ristic, E. M. Stephenson, P. K. Hildebrandt, and D. L. Huxsoll.** 1978. Platelet migration inhibition as an indicator of immunologically mediated target cell injury in canine ehrlichiosis. *Infect. Immun.* **20**:242-247.
14. **Nyindo, M. B. A., M. Ristic, D. L. Huxsoll, and A. R. Smith.** 1971. Tropical canine pancytopenia, *in vitro* cultivation of the causative agent--*Ehrlichia canis*. *Am. J. Vet. Res.* **32**:1651-1658.
15. **Nyindo, M. B. A.** 1975. Immune responses to *Ehrlichia canis* and *Ehrlichia equi* in experimentally infected dogs and ponies. *Ph.D Thesis*, University of Illinois, Urbana, IL.
16. **Ristic, M., D. L. Huxsoll, R. M. Weisiger, P. K. Hildebrandt, and M. B. A. Nyindo.** 1972. Serological diagnosis of tropical canine pancytopenia by indirect fluorescence. *Infect. Immun.* **6**:226-231.
17. **Smith, R. D. and I. Kakoma.** 1986. Computer simulation of platelet kinetics in canine ehrlichiosis, pp. 213-216, *In*: Microbiology 1986. L. Leive (Ed.), ASM Publications, Washington, D.C.
18. **Smith, R. D., J. J. B. Anderson, M. Ristic, and D. L. Huxsoll.** 1972. The use of cerenkov radiation in ^{32}P-labelled platelet survival studies. *Int. J. Appl. Rad. Isotop.* **23**:513-517.
19. **Smith, R. D., J. E. Hooks, D. L. Huxsoll, and M. Ristic.** 1974. Canine ehrlichiosis (tropical canine pancytopenia): survival of phosphorus-32-labeled blood platelets in normal and infected dogs. *Am. J. Vet. Res.* **35**:269-273.
20. **Smith, R. D., M. Ristic, D. L. Huxsoll, and R. A. Baylor.** 1975. Platelet kinetics in canine ehrlichiosis: evidence for increased platelet destruction as the cause of thrombocytopenia. *Infect. Immun.* **11**:1216-1221.
21. **Weisiger, R. M., M. Ristic, and D. L. Huxsoll.** 1975. Kinetics of antibody response to *Ehrlichia canis* assayed by the indirect fluorescent antibody method. *Am. J. Vet. Rest.* **36**:689-694.
22. **Wilkins, R. J., A. I. Hurwitz, and W. J. Dodds-Laffin.** 1973. Immunologically mediated thrombocytopenia in the dog. *J. Am. Vet. Med. Assoc.* **163**:277-282.
23. **van Heerden, J.** 1982. A retrospective study on 120 natural cases of canine ehrlichiosis. *J. S. Afr. Vet. Assoc.* **53**:17-20.

8. EXPERIMENTAL EHRLICHIOSIS IN NONHUMAN PRIMATES

EDWARD H. STEPHENSON, D.V.M., Ph.D.

Abstract

Ehrlichia sennetsu, a recognized human pathogen, has been shown to induce infections in rhesus macaques (*Macaca mulatta*) and cynomolgus macaques (*Macaca fasicularis*). The infections could be initiated by intravenous, intraperitoneal, or subcutaneous inoculation, but not by oral administration. Typically, the monkeys developed a clinical syndrome characterized by mild lymphadenopathy and lethargy lasting 24 to 48 hours. A transient leukocytosis occurred in an occasional monkey 21 to 28 days after inoculation; serum chemistry alterations were limited to increases in serum glucose and haptoglobin, indicative of an ongoing inflammatory response. *Ehrlichemia*, as evidenced by light microscopy of microorganisms in intracytoplasmic inclusions, termed morulae, in circulating monocytes, persisted from 6 to 25 days; and the microorganism was reisolated during the ehrlichemic stage. Challenged monkeys became seropositive by day 12. Cross-reactivity was detected with *E. risticii*, but the predominating serological response was to *E. sennetsu*.

When rhesus macaques were inoculated intravenously with *E. risticii*, the causative agent of equine monocytic ehrlichiosis (syn. Potomac horse fever), the disease induced was analogous to that caused by *E. sennetsu*. Rhesus macaques and baboons (*Papio anubis*) have been successfully infected with *E. equi*, the causative agent of equine ehrlichiosis. Experimental infection of rhesus macaques with *E. bovis* also has been reported and the infectivity of *E. sennetsu* for humans is fully recognized. Susceptibility of nonhuman primates to infection with *E. risticii* and *E. equi* provides a definite basis for consideration for the potential transmission of these ehrlichial agents to man. Additional studies are required for *E. canis* and *E. bovis* before speculations on transmission to man can be substantiated.

Introduction

Initial studies on the susceptibility of nonhuman primates to pathogenic microorganisms typically are designed to provide an indication of the zoonotic potential of a given microorganism. Additionally, when non-human primates are shown to be capable of supporting an infection by a microorganism, a host-parasite model then is available that more closely simulates a human-parasite relationship. It was understandable, therefore, that several investigative teams, over time, evaluated the pathogenesis and immunogenesis of experimentally induced ehrlichial infections in nonhuman primates.

J. C. Williams and I. Kakoma (eds.), Ehrlichiosis, 93–99.

The establishment of the zoonotic potential of the various species of *Ehrlichia* was further enhanced recently. Ehrlichial infections in humans, as evidenced by seroconversion, apparently were induced by *Ehrlichia sp.* other than *E. sennetsu* [15]. This review will attempt to bring together the old and the new facts on the pathogenic potential of ehrlichiae for nonhuman primates.

Ehrlichia sennetsu

Ehrlichia sennetsu is a known human pathogen, having been isolated in 1954 from human cases of sennetsu fever [5,16]. The "mononucleosis-like" disease syndrome in man typically was mild; clinical signs included malaise and headache, lumbago, anorexia, sleeplessness, drenching sweat, constipation, lymphadenopathy, and mild fever. More recent human infections occurring in Malaysia, however, were more severe, with death resulting in several cases (G. E. Lewis, Personal Communication). Epidemiology of the disease in humans still has not been defined.

The early studies of experimental infection of non-huamn primates with *E. sennetsu* used the cynomolgus monkey (*Macaca fasicularis*) as the model [18-21]. Infections could be induced by intraperitoneal or subcutaneous injection of infectious blood or lymph node homogenates, but were not established after oral administration. The rhesus macaque (*Macaca mulatta*), more recently [24], also was shown to be susceptible to experimental infection; infection in these monkeys was induced by intravenous injection of partially purified tissue culture-propagated ehrlichiae of both the Miyayama strain (prototype Japan isolate) and an isolate from Malaysia.

The clinical signs evidenced by the cynomolgus and rhesus macaques, regardless of the route of inoculation, were essentially identical. Typically, the syndrome was characterized by lethargy that occurred 12 to 17 days after inoculation, but abated after 24 to 48 hours, and by development of mild lymphadenopathy. Axillary, and occasionally inguinal, lymph nodes became detectably enlarged by day 15 after inoculation and remained moderately enlarged throughout 60 days of observation. The monkeys inoculated with the Malaysian isolate exhibited the greatest response. Fulminant infections did not occur in either species of monkey.

An absolute lymphocytosis occurred in challenged monkeys during the acute infection, and a transient leukocytosis developed in an occasional monkey 21 to 28 days after infection. Serum chemistry alterations were limited to increases in serum glucose and haptoglobin, which are indicative of ongoing inflammatory responses. Gross or histologic pathological alterations were not observed in any monkey after the acute infection period.

Definitive confirmation of infection was achieved by visualization of the ehrlichial intracytoplasmic inclusions in the peripheral circulating monocytes, reisolation of the microorganisms from the blood of infected monkeys, and demonstration of specific humoral antibody response. Infected rhesus macaques became seropositive by day 12 after inoculation. Although there was a cross-reactivity with *E. risticii*, the predominating serological response was to the challenge isolate of *E. sennetsu*.

Ehrlichia risticii

The causative agent of Potomac horse fever was shown in 1985 to be an ehrlichia [9], and was subsequently named *E. risticii* [10]. This microorganism is serologically related to *E. sennetsu*; therefore, it was of interest to evaluate the zoonotic potential of this microorganism [24]. In the event that *E. risticii* is a zoonotic agent, the close association of equids and humans suggested the possible transmission and the development of an epidemic in humans.

Studies in rhesus macaques inoculated intravenously with *E. risticii* produced a clinical syndrome which was indistinguishable from that caused by *E. sennetsu*. Each of the monkeys became detectably ill with a mild clinically recognized disease. Lymphadenopathy was evidenced in two monkeys by day 15, but was delayed until day 32 for the third monkey. A mild absolute lymphocytosis was the only alteration noted among the hematologic parameters. Elevated serum glucose concentrations indicated the ongoing inflammatory response after infection. No gross or histologic lesions related to ehrlichial infection were identified.

A positive humoral antibody response developed that was principally against *E. risticii*, the challenge ehrlichia, although there was a cross-reactivity to *E. sennetsu*. Again, confirmation was attained by visualization of intracytoplasmic inclusions in circulating monocytes and by reisolation of the challenge ehrlichiae from the peripheral blood monocytes.

Ehrlichia equi

Equine ehrlichiosis induced by *E. equi* primarily has been recognized in the Sacramento Valley in California [6,23]. This ehrlichia has exhibited a broad experimental host range, which includes the horse, pony, burro, goat, sheep, dog, cat, and non-huamn primates [13,23]. Both rhesus macaques and baboons (*Papio anubis*) were successfully infected with *E. equi* after intravenous inoculation of whole blood collected from horses in the acute phase of infection. The disease produced was inapparent. There were no significant changes in clinical behavior, appetite, or physical condition. Morulae were visualized in the circulating neutrophilis, accompanied by pyrexia, increased sedimentation rate, and mild anemia. All clinicopathologic parameters returned to baseline within 7 days of the disappearance of morulae. Gross or histologic alterations attributable to *E. equi* infection were not observed. Inoculation of a susceptible horse with pooled blood from two infected rhesus macaques induced severe clinical signs of equine ehrlichiosis, thus showing virulence for equids had not diminished with passage in nonhuman primates.

A specific immune response follows infection of nonhuman primates with *E. equi*. When convalescent monkeys were challenged with *E. equi*-

infected blood, they were resistant, indicating a protective immune status had been established [12].

Ehrlichia canis

Ehrlichia canis, the type species for the genus, undoubtedly has been studied more than any of the other species within the genus. To date, the vertebrate hosts for *E. canis* have been restricted to members of the family *Canidae* [1,4,11,17]. Among dogs and other canidae, the acute phase of infection commonly is followed by an inapparent (mild chronic) infection in which there is a gradual return of clinicopathologic parameters to normal values even though the animals remain infected. In a few animals, however, the disease progresses to a fulminant stage, referred to as the severe chronic form.

Donatien and Lestoquard [2] reported the successful infection of a single *Macaca sylvana* (*inuus*) after the injection of emulsions of *R. sanguineus* larvae from a female tick that had engorged on a dog in the acute phase of canine ehrlichiosis. Confirmation of these findings has yet to be attained. Experimental inoculation of *Macaca mulatta* with *E. canis*-infected canine monocyte cultures did not yield any evidence of survival, growth, or multiplication of ehrlichiae in any of six inoculated monkeys [14]. No alterations in the clinical status or clinicopathologic parameters were detected. Further, it now has been substantiated that transovarial transmission of *E. canis* from adult female to larval ticks does not occur [7,22]. It would appear, therefore, that rhesus macaques are not suitable experimental models and are highly unlikely to be natural reservoirs of *E. canis*.

Ehrlichia bovis

Ehrlichia bovis, comparable to *E. canis*, was reported to infect *Macaca sylvana* (*inuus*) [3]. A single monkey was inoculated with blood from a bovine with a mixed infection of theileria and *E. bovis*. The monkey subsequently exhibited morulae in the peripheral circulating monocytes, developed pyrexia, and became lethargic. However, it cannot be ascertained from the reported data whether the clinical responses were induced by the ehrlichiae or by the theileria. Further studies with *E. bovis* have yet to be performed which would substantiate or repudiate the observations of Donatien and Lestoguard.

Conclusion

Studies on the susceptibility of nonhuman primates with several species of *Ehrlichia* have been performed by several investigative teams. Such studies provide an indication of the zoonotic potential of a microorganism, plus establish whether the nonhuman primate can be used as an animal model to study the pathogenesis and immunogenesis of the agent.

Ehrlichia sennetsu, a recognized human pathogen has been shown to induce infections in rhesus macaques (*Macaca mulatta*) and cynomolgus macaques (*Macaca fasicularis*). The infections could be initiated by intravenous, intraperitoneal, or subcutaneous inoculation, but not via oral administration. Typically, the monkeys developed a clinical syndrome characterized by lethargy that abated after 24 to 48 hours, and by development of mild lymphadenopathy. A transient leukocytosis occurred in an occasional monkey 21 to 28 days after inoculation; serum chemistry alterations were limited to increases in serum glucose and haptoglobin, indicative of an ongoing inflammatory response. Gross or histologic alterations could not be detected after the acute infection period. Ehrlichemia, as evidenced by observation of intracytoplasmic inclusions (morulae) in circulating monocytes, persisted from day 6 to 25; reisolation of the challenge microorganism was accomplished during the ehrlichemic stage. Challenged monkeys became seropositive by day 12. Cross-reactivity was detected with *E. risticii*, but the predominating serological response was to *E. sennetsu*.

When rhesus macaques were inoculated intravenously with *E. risticii*, the causative agent of Potomac horse fever or equine monocytic ehrlichiosis, the disease induced was analogous to that caused by *E. sennetsu*. Rhesus macaques and baboons (*Pabio anubis*) have been successfully infected with *E. equi*, the causative agent of equine ehrlichiosis. Clinical alterations were limited to pyrexia, morulae in the circulating granulocytes, and a transient increase in sedimentation rate accompanied by mild anemia. Donatien and Lestoguard, in 1937, reported the successful infection of a single *Macaca sylvana* (*inuus*) with *E. canis*. These early observations, however, could not be confirmed. Evidence has not been obtained for the survival, growth, or multiplication of *E. canis*, much less inducement of a clinical syndrome, in monkeys challenged with cell culture-propagated *E. canis*. Experimental infection of rhesus macaques with *E. bovis* also has been reported.

The infectivity of *E. sennetsu* for humans is fully recognized. Susceptibility of nonhuman primates to infection with *E. risticii* and *E. equi* provides a definite basis for consideration of the potential transmission of these ehrlichiae to humans. Additional studies are required for *E. canis* and *E. bovis* before similar considerations of transmission to humans should be contemplated.

The urgency in pursuing the determination of the *E. canis*-primate host relationship is driven by the recent reports of ehrlichiosis in humans. The cases of ehrlichiosis were identified by seroconversion after an acute febrile illness; intracytoplasmic inclusions in circulating monocytes were observed only in the initial reported case, and an ehrlichial isolate has yet to be obtained. Recently, however, it was reported that *E. canis* could be adapted to replicate in primary cultures of human monocytes [8]. The rate of infection initially was slow, but was enhanced with time to yield a high percentage of *in-vitro* infected cells, each containing typical intracytoplasmic inclusions.

Literature Cited

1. **Amyx, H. L., and D. L. Huxsoll.** 1973. Red and gray foxes - potential reservoir hosts for *Ehrlichia canis*. *J. Wildl. Dis.* **9**:47-50.

2. **Donatien, A., and F. Lestoquard.** 1937. État actuel des connaissances sur les rickettsioses animales. *Arch. Inst. Pasteur Algérie.* **15**:142-187.
3. **Donatien, A., and F. Lestoquard.** 1940. Rickettsiose bovine Algérienne a *R. bovis. Bull. Soc. Pathol. Exot. Filiales.* **31**:245-248.
4. **Ewing, S. A., R. G. Buckner, and B. G. Stringer.** 1964. The coyote, a potential host for *Babesia canis* and *Ehrlichia sp. J. Parasitol.* **50**:704.
5. **Fukuda, T., Y. Kada, and T. Kitao.** 1954. Studies on causative agent of "Hyuganetsu" disease. I. Isolation of the agent and its inoculation trial in human beings. *J. Med. Biol.* **32**:200-209.
6. **Gribble, D. H.** 1969. Equine ehrlichiosis. *J. Am. Vet. Med. Assoc.* **155**:462-469.
7. **Groves, M. G., G. L. Dennis, H. L. Amyx, and D. L. Huxsoll.** 1975. Transmission of *Ehrlichia canis* to dogs by ticks (*Rhipicephalus sanguineus*). *Am. J. Vet. Res.* **36**:937-940.
8. **Holland, C. J., I. Kakoma, and M. Ristic.** 1988 (Abstract). Adaptation of *Ehrlichia canis* to growth in primary human monocyte cell cultures. *Proceedings of Ann. Meet. Am. Soc. Trop. Med. Hyg.* **37**:168.
9. **Holland, C. J., M. Ristic, A. I. Cole, P. Johnson, G. Baker, and T. Goetz.** 1985. Isolation, experimental transmission, and characterization of causative agent of Potomac horse fever. *Science* **227**:522-524.
10. **Holland, C. J., E. Weiss, W. Burgdorfer, A. I. Cole, and I. Kakoma.** 1985. *Ehrlichia risticii* sp. nov.: etiologic agent of equine monocytic ehrlichiosis (synonym, Potomac horse fever). *Intl. J. Syst. Bacteriol.* **35**:524-526.
11. **Huxsoll, D. L.** 1976. Canine ehrlichiosis (tropical canine pancytopenia): a review. *Vet. Parasitol.* **2**:49-60.
12. **Lewis, G. E., Jr.** 1976. Equine ehrlichiosis: a comparison between *E. equi* and other pathogenic species of *Ehrlichia. Vet. Parasitol.* **2**:61-74.
13. **Lewis, G. E., Jr., D. L. Huxsoll, M. Ristic, and A. J. Johnson.** 1975. Experimentally induced infection of dogs, cats, and nonhuman primates with *Ehrlichia equi*, etiologic agent of equine ehrlichiosis. *Am. J. Vet. Res.* **36**:85-88.
14. **Lewis, G., D. Renquist, I. Hemelt, D. Huxsoll, M. Ristic, and E. H. Stephenson.** 1975. Experimental inoculation of *Macaca mulatta* with *Ehrlichia canis*-infected canine monocyte cell culture, pp. 15. *Proc. 56th Ann. Meet. Conf. Res. Workers Animal Dis.* Chicago, IL.
15. **Maeda, K., N. Markowitz, R. C. Hawley, M. Ristic, D. Cox, and J. E. McDade.** 1987. Human infection with *Ehrlichia canis*, a leukocytic rickettsia. *N. Eng. J. Med.* **316**:853-856.
16. **Misao, T., and Y. Kobayashi.** 1954. Studies on infectious mononucleosis. I. On the isolation of the causative agent from blood, bone marrow and lymph gland with mice. *Tokyo Med. J.* **71**:683-686.
17. **Neitz, W. O., and A. D. Thomas.** 1938. Rickettsiosis in the dog. *J. S. Afr. Vet. Med. Assoc.* **9**:166-174.

18. **Ohtaki, S., and A. Shishido.** 1965. Studies on infectious mononucleosis induced in the monkey by experimental infection with *Rickettsia sennetsu*. II. Pathological findings. *Jap. J. Med. Sci. Biol.* **18**:85-99.
19. **Ohtawara, T., Y. Takayama, I. Honda, S. Yamanouchi, and T. Nishikame.** 1943. Studies on endemic glandular fever. Experimental inoculation of the agent of endemic glandular fever into monkeys and human volunteers. *Nippon Igaku Kenko Hoken.* **3337**:1076-1081.
20. **Sato, K., T. Ohtawara, T. Yamada, and H. Kataoka.** 1925. Studies on endemic glandular fever. *J. Kmamoto Med. Soc.* **1**:14-22.
21. **Shishido, A., S. Honjo, M. Suganuma, S. Ohtaki, M. Hikita, T. Fujiwara, and M. Takasaka.** 1965. Studies on infectious mononucleosis induced in the monkey by experimental infection with *Rickettsia sennetsu*. I. Clinical observations and etiological investigations. *Jap. J. Med. Sci. Biol.* **18**:73-83.
22. **Smith, R. D., and M. Ristic.** 1977. Ehrlichiae, pp. 295-328, *In* J. P. Kreier (ed.), Parasitic protozoa, Vol. IV. Academic Press, New York.
23. **Smith, R. D., D. M. Sells, E. H. Stephenson, M. Ristic, and D. L. Huxsoll.** 1976. Development of *Ehrlichia canis*, causative agent of canine ehrlichiosis, in the tick *Rhipicephalus sanguineus* and its differentiation from a symbiotic rickettsia. *Am. J. Vet. Res.* **37**:119-126.
24. **Stannard, A. A., D. H. Gribble, and R. S. Smith.** 1969. Equine ehrlichiosis: a disease with similarities to tick-borne fever and bovine petechial fever. *Vet. Rec.* **84**:149-150.
25. **Stephenson, E. H., A. D. King, R. B. Moeller, J. C. Williams, C. J. Holland, and M. Ristic.** 1989. Pathophysiology of *Ehrlichia risticii*, causative agent of Potomac horse fever, and *Ehrlichia sennetsu* in rhesus macaques (*Macaca mulatta*). In Press.

9. HUMAN EHRLICHIOSIS IN THE UNITED STATES

DANIEL B. FISHBEIN, M.D.

Abstract

In 1986, a 51-year-old man hospitalized with an illness clinically resembling "spotless" Rocky Mountain spotted fever was shown to have ehrlichiosis. Subsequently, 100 additional cases among patients in 15 states have been identified by various investigators. Most patients had a recent tick exposure, and acute febrile illness with nonspecific symptoms and mild degrees of liver dysfunction, leukopenia, and thrombocytopenia. Intraleukocytic inclusions have been found in only three cases. Active surveillance in hospitalized patients in Georgia revealed a rate of 5.3 per 100,000 population. Cases differed from the noncases in that they were more likely to report a recent tick bite ($P < 0.02$) and reside in a rural county ($P < 0.02$). Cases also had lower white blood cell counts ($P < 0.001$), platelet counts ($P = 0.01$), and higher aspartate aminotransferase ($P < 0.005$) and alanine aminotransferase ($P < 0.01$) levels at the time of admission to the hospital. Ehrlichiosis is an important cause of acute febrile illness in some parts of the United States, and is distinguishable from other febrile illnesses, primarily by history of tick bite and the presence of abnormal hematology and liver function test results. The putative etiologic agent has not been isolated, but is considered to be closely related to *E. canis*. The possibility of the zooanthropozoonotic nature of erlichiosis is discussed but remains largely speculative and epidemiologically unsubstantiated. The differential diagnosis of ehrlichiosis-like disease and Rocky Mountain spotted fever (without a rash) is discussed and criteria for ehrlichiosis case definition are suggested.

Introduction

In 1986, five rickettsial diseases were considered indigenous to the United States. Recognized in the beginning of the 20th century, Rocky Mountain spotted fever (RMSF) was endemic in the late 1980s in most states along the eastern seaboard in the south central part of the country [4] with 500-600 cases reported each year. Q fever was less common than Rocky Mountain spotted fever, with less than 100 widely distributed cases reported each year [18-19]. Sporadic typhus, associated with flying squirrels, was a winter disease; only a few cases were recognized annually [13]. Endemic or flea-borne typhus was found in areas of lower socioeconomic status in southern Texas, California, and Hawaii [21]. Rickettsialpox was occasionally recognized in New York City [1].

J. C. Williams and I. Kakoma (eds.), Ehrlichiosis, 100–111.

Ehrlichia canis, the type species of the genus Ehrlichia (Table 1), has long been recognized to cause acute and chronic disease in dogs worldwide [2, 6, 11, 16]. However, before the report discussed below, *E. sennetsu* was the only species of this genus that had been recognized as causing human disease [20].

TABLE 1. Taxonomy of the ehrlichia, and the diseases caused by individual species.

Order:	Rickettsiales
Family:	Rickettsiaceae
Tribe:	Ehrlichiae
Genus:	Ehrlichia
Species (disease):	
E. canis* (Canine ehrlichiosis)	
E. sennetsu (Sennetsu fever)	
E. risticii (Potomac horse fever)	
E. equi (Equine ehrlichiosis)	
E. phagocytophila (Tick-borne fever in sheep)	
Species incertae:	
E. bovis	
E. platys (Infectious cyclic thrombocytopenia in dogs)	
E. ovina	
E. Kurlovi	

* Type species.

Recognition of Human Ehrlichiosis in the United States

Only 25% of sera from patients suspected of RMSF reveal diagnoses titers with specific serological testing [24]. Typical of patients suspected of having RMSF without serological evidence of the disease was a 51-year-old black male from Detroit [12]. In March, 1986, he was vacationing with his family, planting trees on some property that he owned in central Arkansas. A few hours later, he noticed some ticks attached to his neck and removed them. Ten days later, after returning to Detroit, the patient developed a low-grade fever, muscle aches, and myalgia. He sought medical care at a number of hospital emergency rooms in the area; no cause for his illness could be determined and he was sent home. Finally, on April 14, 16 days after the tick bites, his condition had deteriorated to the point that he was admitted to Henry Ford Hospital. His temperature was 40°C, and he presented with rigors, headaches, and was confused. His physical examination was normal but laboratory evaluation revealed a white blood cell count of 4600/mm^3, thrombocytopenia (platelet count of 18000/mm^3), and evidence of disseminated intravascular coagulation. Liver function tests were also abnormal, with a serum glutamic oxaloacetic transaminase (SGOTase) of 768 IU/L, a serum glutamic pyruvic transaminase (SGPTase) of 403 IU/L, alkaline phosphatase of 173 IU/L, and bilirubin which rose to 5 mg/dL. The hemoglobin level fell from 12.6 g/dL to 7.9 g/dL, and the creatinine level rose to 9.6 ml/dL, necessitating hemodialysis. Because of the confusion, a computerized tomography scan of the head was undertaken, but this examination was normal. Lumbar puncture revealed no pleocytosis, but the protein was elevated to 70 mg/dL.

At this point, the differential diagnosis included RMSF without a rash, leptospirosis, and tularemia; the patient was initially treated with chloramphenicol. Unusual inclusions in the patients mononuclear cells were noted by one of the interns at the hospital. Although these inclusions were inititally thought to be Döhle's bodies (small coccus-shaped bodies occurring in the polynuclear leukocytes in several diseases, especially scarlet fever), the young doctor pointed them out to a hematopathologist, Dr. Koishi Maeda, who recognized them as unusual and obtained buffy coat specimens from the patient. These were processed for electron microscopy and revealed microorganisms in the white cells. Therapy with chloramphenicol was begun; the treatment was later switched to tetracycline and the patient recovered after a stormy course complicated by disseminated candidiasis.

When serological tests were negative for a number of infectious diseases, Dr. Maeda contacted Dr. Joseph McDade, a microbiologist at the Centers for Disease Control (CDC), who helped identify the inclusions. Although the indirect immunofluorescent antibody (IFA) test was negative for *Rickettsia rickettsii*, the clinical response to tetracycline and the history of the tick bite convinced the doctors at Henry Ford Hospital that they were dealing with RMSF. Dr. McDade suspected otherwise; he recognized that the inclusions resembled *Ehrlichia* and, after consulting with pathologists at CDC, he contacted various experts around the country to arrange for serological testing for the various *Ehrlichia* species. This testing was eventually undertaken by Jacqueline Dawson in the laboratory of Miodrag Ristic at the University of Illinois and revealed a reciprocal (titer) of 640 to *E. canis*; the titer fell to 40 four months later. Although titers to the other ehrlichiae species were also somewhat elevated, they were considerably lower. The inclusions and the serological data provided sufficient evidence for this to be considered the first case of human infection with an *Ehrlichia* in the United States [12]. What remained unknown was the species of this ehrlichia and its place in the genus.

Initial Surveillance for Ehrlichiosis in Humans in the United States

One of the first tasks was to determine the background distribution of antibody titers to *E. canis* in humans. Investigators at the CDC and at the Oklahoma State Health Department attempted to determine if other patients in the United States initially suspected of having RMSF or other tick-borne diseases might have had an infection with an ehrlichia [8, 17]. Dr. Leigh Sawyer and I therefore conducted a serosurvey among employees of a log mill a few hundred yards away from the place where the index case [12] had apparently been exposed. For comparison, Dr. Sawyer obtained sera from employees of the Arkansas State Health Department, most of whom were rarely, if ever, exposed to ticks. Only three of the 84 persons had titers to *E. canis* >40 and none were >80. Moreover, there was no significant difference in the distribution of titers among the loggers and health department employees, suggesting that these low titers were non-specific and did not reflect infection with an ehrlichia. We therefore decided that a fourfold rise or fall in titer and a minimum titer of 80, should be required to define a case.

We tested paired serum specimens that had been submitted to CDC or state health departments for RMSF, Lyme disease, Colorado tick fever, and other zoonoses. These specimens were tested in an IFA test using an *E. canis* antigen maintained in continous culture at the University of Illinois or ProtaTek, Minneapolis, MN [16]. Among the first cases recognized were those reported by Jeffery Taylor [21] of the Texas Department of Health. Of particular interest were the extremes of illness noted in this report: One woman was so severely ill that she required intensive care and multiple transfusions [21]; another woman had absolutely no symptoms, perhaps because her physician treated her prophylactically with tetracycline.

Dr. Thomas Eng with CDC compiled data on cases recognized through May 1988 [3]. At that time, 46 human cases of ehrlichiosis had been diagnosed in 13 states. Patients were presumed to have been exposed in their state of residence, unless conflicting information and exposure to ticks in another state was available. Many characteristics of the initial cases were detected in subsequent cases (Table 2). Virtually all patients had a fever and many reported headaches, anorexia, myalgia, rigors or chills, nausea or vomiting, and weight loss. A rash, absent in the initial case, infrequently accompanied this disease, in contrast to RMSF. Laboratory evaluation of the initial 46 patients revealed that slightly over half had leukopenia and thrombocytopenia and more than three-quarters had elevated hepatic transaminase levels.

TABLE 2. Clinical and laboratory findings commonly observed in human ehrlichiosis patients.

Sign or Symptom	Percent	Laboratory findings	Percent
Fever	96	Leukopenia	61
Headache	80	Thrombocytopenia	52
Anorexia	79		
Myalgia	74	Elevated APATase[a]	76
Chills/rigors	70	Elevated ALATase[b]	75
Nausea/Vomiting	69	Elevated ALKPase[c]	50
Weight loss	60	Elevated bilirubin[d]	29
Rash	20		

[a]APATase = aspartate aminotransferase; [b]ALATase = alanine aminotransferase; [c]ALKPase = alkaline phosphatase; [d]total bilirubin.

Although patients with ehrlichiosis were, in general, somewhat older than those with RMSF, cases were sometimes noted in younger groups. The first pediatric cases were reported by Dr. Morven Edwards from Baylor [5]. Interestingly, one of these children had a rash on the palms and soles that appeared similar to RMSF. Subsequently, a number of other pediatric cases have been reported. Also of interest were the limited findings suggesting the pathogenesis of the hematologic abnormalities. A few patients had bone marrow examinations because of unexplained hematologic abnormalities. Most patients had normal marrow examinations [7, 9]; however, a few had hypoplasia [14], with peripheral destruction or sequestration as the etiology of the leukopenia and thrombocytopenia, suggesting the human agent supressed the bone marrow, as well.

The question remained whether the clinical and epidemiological features of these initial cases were truly representative. Because these initial cases had largely been ascertained among patients (initially) suspected of having RMSF or other tick-borne diseases, we wondered if other forms of the disease might be obscured by clinical presentations that did not suggest RMSF. The initial clue that there were other forms of the disease came from one of the patients in the surveillance discussed above [3].

An Outbreak of Human Ehrlichiosis [15]

In January 1987, as part of the retrospective serosurvey discussed above, 47 sera were obtained from the Connecticut State Health Department. About half of these sera had initially been submitted to the health department for *Borrelia burgdorferi* serology, and the other half had been submitted for *R. rickettsii* serology. Testing of these 47 specimens revealed one patient who seroconverted to *E. canis*. To our surprise, acute serum had been obtained in July of 1985, almost a year before the case identified by Dr. Maeda. The patient's titer rose from 20 to 2560 over 12 days between July 23, 1985 and August 4, 1985. Titers in the other 46 patients from this state health laboratory were all less than 80 in both sera.

The patient, a 40-year-old Army reservist sought medical care from his private physician on July 20, 1985, because of a 3- day history of fever, chills, myalgia, headaches, and mild nausea. Physical examination was normal and there was no rash. Physical examination revealed a temperature of only 100.2°F. Because of the suspicion of Lyme disease, the patient was treated with penicillin 250 mg, four times a day. On July 23, 1985, 3 days later, the patient was no better. His temperature had risen to 101°F and laboratory studies were undertaken. He was found to have a hematocrit of 47.3% but his white blood cell count was only 2800/mm^3. A platelet estimate was normal. His physician increased his penicillin to 500 mg four times a day and ordered serological testing for a number tick-borne agents. This revealed a slight titer rise to *B. burgdorferi* and negative serology to other tick-borne agents. His serum was, therefore, among those forwarded to the Centers for Disease Control for ehrlichia testing.

Discussions with the patient and subsequently with Dr. Lyle Peterson, a CDC Epidemiology Intelligence Service Officer assigned to the Connecticut State Health Department, revealed that the patient was one of 106 United States Army reservists who went on active duty at Fort Monmouth, New Jersey, on June 30, 1985. During the first week, the unit camped and conducted field exercises in an underdeveloped area with knee-high grass and brush, and many ticks. Between July 5 and July 12, 1985, three reservists developed erythema migrans, the pathognomonic rash of Lyme disease. The other reservists were informed about Lyme disease and instructed to seek medical care if symptoms developed. At the same time, the EPICON Unit at Walter Reed was contacted and an investigation was begun. On August 11, 1985, 5 weeks after the exercise, EPICON reconvened the unit to investigate the possible Lyme disease outbreak; the investigators indeed found that other reservists had become ill. Questionnaires were administered and serum specimens were drawn from the 75 reservists who had participated in the training in New Jersey as well as 12 reservists who had attended the exercises.

The army reserve unit was reconvened on December 7, 1985, about 6 months after the exposure to ticks. A second questionnaire was administered, and a second serum specimen collected. Unfortunately, the initial investigation was inconclusive; there was no clear relationship between clinical illness and antibody titers to *B. burgdorferi*. Almost 2 years later, these same sera were analyzed at CDC which found that many of the reservists had titers $\geq$80 to *E. canis*, but few had evidence of rising or falling titers. The lack of fluctuation in titers was believed due to the late collection of acute sera (5 weeks after exposure). We therefore defined the case as a reservist with a single titer of $\geq$ 160 to *E. canis* at the time of either the August or December blood drawing.

By using this definition, nine (12%) of the 74 trainees had evidence of an infection with an ehrlichia. None of the 12 who did not attend the field exercises in New Jersey had evidence of infection. Demographic and epidemiological characteristics of patients who met the case definition and those who did not were similar. The median age of cases was 40 years; the median age of noncases was 35 years. Their race, sex, number of years in the reserve, number of training activities in which they participated, and exposure to outdoor areas prior to the reserve exercises were similar. The proportion of reservists in the two groups that used tick repellents during training was similar. Although 100% of the case reservists and 77% of the noncase reservists reported tick bites, this difference was not statistically significant. The cases were somewhat more likely to have missed more than 1 day of work because of an illness that developed after the tick bites. In fact, three of the cases (33%) and only four (7%) of the noncases missed 1 day of work. Seven (78%) of the cases sought medical care in the month after their tick exposure, while only 10 (16%) of the noncases did so. No patient in either group was hospitalized. Cases were also more likely to report certain symptoms, specifically arthralgia, myalgia, headaches, and anorexia. Unfortunately, because fever was not among the questions on the original questionnaire, we do not know how the two groups differed in this regard. However, all of the three reservists who had a white blood cell count obtained because of their illnesses had evidence of leukopenia (less than 4000 cells/mm^3). All the reservists recovered without complications. Altogether seven of the case reservists were mildly ill, two were entirely asymptomatic.

Differential Characteristics of Rocky Mountain Spotted Fever and Human Ehrlichiosis in Oklahoma

To elucidate further the epidemiology of human ehrlichiosis, and to help clarify the differences between ehrlichiosis and RMSF, Harkess *et al.*, [10] from the Oklahoma State Health Department tested all patients with suspected tick-borne diseases from whom paired serum specimens were submitted for antibodies to either *E. canis* or *R. rickettsii* [9,10]. Remarkably, the number of sera indicating recent infection with an ehrlichia and the number indicating recent infection with *R. rickettsii* was identical: 29 (12%) of 249 paired sera submitted showed evidence of recent infection with *E. canis*, while an equal number had a recent infection with *R. rickettsii*, and the remaining 191 were seronegative for both agents. Some of the features which distinguished these three groups of patients are shown in Table 3.

TABLE 3. Clinical, laboratory, and epidemiologic features of patients with serological evidence of infection with *R. rickettsii* and *E. canis*-like microorganisms, and controls; Oklahoma, 1987 [10].

Sign or symptom	Infecting Agent		
	Ehrlichia canis	*Rickettsia rickettsii*	Neither
Fever (>38°C)	85%	96%	77%
Headache	85	95	79
Myalgia	82	82	74
Nausea/vomiting	42	76*	53
Rash: any	35	83*	50
Rash: palm/soles	8	62*	26
Hospitalized	38	62	36
White blood cells[a]	38%	13%*	11%*
Platelet count[b]	47	52	13*
Tick bite	74	76	52
Tick Exposure	81	84	58*
Mosquito bite	48	52	55
Chigger bite	41	30	31
Owned dog	63	92*	75
Owned cat	41	36	40

[a]<4200/cubic mm.
[b]<150,000/cubic mm.
*Significant difference versus patients with evidence of *E. canis*-like infection.

Patients with ehrlichiosis were somewhat older (mean 36.7 years) than patients with RMSF (21.6 years). Only 38% of patients with ehrlichiosis were hospitalized, compared to 62% of those with RMSF. Although fever, headache, myalgia, and nausea and vomiting were reported by more than 80% of patients in both groups, nausea or vomiting and rash were significantly more common in patients with RMSF. Leukopenia (<4200 WBC/mm^3) was reported in 38% of patients with ehrlichiosis, versus only 13% of those with RMSF, but thrombocytopenia was found in about 50% of patients with either disease.

A range of specific and non-specific disease syndromes and malignancies including those of known etiology have to be considered in the differential diagnosis of human ehrlichiosis (Table 4). Noteworthy is the important distinction betwen RMSF and ehrlichiosis.

Table 4. Differential Diagnosis of Human Ehrlichiosis.

Tick borne diseases	Other diseases
Rocky Mountain spotted fever	Pyelonephritis
Tularemia	Prostatitis
Relapsing fever	Non-A non-B hepatitis
Lyme disease	Gastroenteritis
Colorado tick fever	Q fever
Babesiosis	Hematologic malignancies[a]

[a]With leukopenia or thrombocytopenia.

Active Surveillance of Human Ehrlichiosis in Southeast Georgia [7]

The studies of human ehrlichiosis previously discussed were largely based on paired sera submitted by physicians to state health departments because of suspicion of a tick-bone disease, usually RMSF. Many physicians choose only to pursue a serodiagnosis when the illness is unusual or especially severe, and, even under these circumstances, many physicians do not pursue serological testing if the patient recovers. We were interested in determining the exact frequency of this illness in a given geographic region. We wanted to avoid the bias introduced by obtaining sera only from patients suspected of having RMSF, a bias which would tend to make the features of ehrlichiosis resemble those of RMSF, i.e., history of tick bite and presence of a rash. We therefore attempted to determine the characteristics of ehrlichiosis in a group of patients hospitalized for fevers of unclear etiology.

We chose the area around Glynn County, Georgia (population 100,000) in the southeast corner of the state, as the site of the study. A single hospital serves the county and surrounding rural areas. In 1985 a physician in Brunswick, the largest city in the county, noted three patients with histories of tick bites and acute febrile illness, leukopenia, thrombocytopenia, and abnormal liver function tests. Although serological testing for RMSF and Q fever were negative, subsequent investigations at the CDC revealed that these patients had human ehrlichiosis [14].

In the prospective study all patients admitted to the hospital between April 1, 1987, and September 30, 1988, were screened for the presence of a fever (temperature > 100° F). We excluded residents of extended care facilities and patients with pneumonia, positive bacterial cultures, surgical conditions, and diseases involving the immune system (HIV infection, chronic renal failure, malignancy) if these conditions were documented within 24 hours of admission. An acute serum specimen was collected from each individual. After discharge, patients were interviewed, convalescent serum specimens were obtained, and hospital records were reviewed. Patients with a fourfold or greater rise or fall in titer to *E. canis* were considered to be cases. In the 18 months of the study, between April 1, 1987, and September 30, 1988, 75 patients were enrolled. Eight (10.5%) fulfilled the serological case definition. The rate of ehrlichiosis in this area was estimated 5.3 per 100,000. Interestingly, during the entire 18 months, only one case of RMSF was detected in this population, in spite of the fact that hospitalized patients with this disease would certainly have been detected by our surveillance system.

The age of case patients was somewhat higher than noncases, but the differences were not statistically significant. However, cases were more likely than noncases to have had an onset of illness in May or June, a tick bite within 28 days of onset of illness, and reported a rural residence defined as outside the city of Brunswick.

Symptoms and signs among the cases and noncases were, in general, quite similar. Although all patients had to have a fever to fulfill criteria for inclusion in the study, case patients had a somewhat higher initial temperature than noncases (102.0^{o} vs. 101.0°F). Rigors, sweating, headaches, myalgia, anorexia, weight loss, nausea were all reported by more than half of the case patients; but the proportion of noncase patients reporting these symptoms was similar. A rash was detected in only one (13%) of the eight case patients and 14 (23%) of the noncases. This suggests that rash is an infrequent feature of human ehrlichiosis and of little use in distinguishing cases from noncases.

Laboratory evaluation of the cases revealed a number of differences between them and the noncases. Although the hematocrits at the time of admission to the hospital were somewhat higher in cases than noncases (42.5% vs. 40%), hematocrits fell to a median 6.6% among cases, with 63% of the cases eventually developing anemia during the course of hospitalization. The fall in hematocrit was significantly greater among cases than noncase patients. Leukopenia was also substantially more frequent in cases than noncases; three (38%) of the eight cases were leukopenic at the time of admission to the hospital. The median white blood cell (WBC) of cases was 4450/mm^3 among cases and 9000/mm^3 in noncases. The WBC fell further in many of the cases, reaching a median low of 3650/mm^3 during hospitalization. Leukopenia was present in six (75%) of the eight cases and only seven (10%) of the noncases. The median platelet count at the time of admission was 133,000 among the cases and 266,000 among the noncases. Like the WBC, the platelet count fell further during the course of hospitalization in the cases than the noncases, reaching a median minimum of 80,000^3 per ml.

Liver function tests were also more frequently abnormal in cases than noncases, although at the time of admission, these abnormalities were relatively mild. The median SGOT of cases at the time of admission was 68 U/L versus 29 U/L among the noncases. Although 88% of the cases had an abnormal SGOT at the time of admission (greater than 35 U/L), 38% of the noncases also had mild abnormalities of their SGOT. However, during the course of hospitalization, SGOT rose to a median of 194 U/L among the cases and only a slight rise to 31 U/L, among the noncases.

Similarly, SGPT was more likely to be abnormal at the time of admission among cases than noncases; the median SGPT at admission among the cases was 62 IU/L and 20 IU/L among the noncases. SGPT rose to a median of 176 IU/L among the cases and only 29 IU/L among the noncases. All these differences were statistically significant. Milder abnormalities, of only borderline significance, were detected in other liver function tests, such as the alkaline phosphatase and bilirubin.

Conclusion

Human ehrlichiosis is a newly recognized bacterial disease which appears to have fairly distinct epidemiological and laboratory characteristics. Results of case-control studies reveal that human ehrlichiosis is associated with tick bites. Based on active surveillance studies in Brunswick, Georgia, human ehrlichiosis is found in areas where RMSF is uncommon. Therefore, in some areas, human ehrlichiosis should be suspected, even if RMSF is not widely recognized. In other parts of the country there may be extensive overlap between these two diseases.

Based on the studies in Georgia, Oklahoma, Texas, and New Jersey, there is a wide range of host responses after infection which vary from asymptomatic infection to a life-threatening or fatal illness [23]. Future directions for this research include continuing surveillance to determine the geographic distribution, case fatality rate, and possibility of chronic human infection. When more specific reagents become available, widespread serodiagnosis should be widely performed in human and animal populations to identify transmission and potential reservoirs of ehrlichiosis. Finally, it is necessary to isolate this agent from a human to determine the exact cause of the human illness and its definitive relationship to the other ehrlichia species.

Literature Cited

1. **Brettman, L. R., S. Lewin, R. S. Holzman, W. D. Goldman, J. S. Marr, P. Kechijian, and R. Schinella.** 1981. Rickettsialpox: report of an outbreak and a contemporary review. *Medicine* **60**:363-372.
2. **Buhles Jr, W. C., D. L. Huxsoll, and M. Ristic.** 1974. Tropical canine pancytopenia: clinical, hematologic, and serological response of dogs to *Ehrlichia canis* infection, tetracycline therapy, and challenge inoculation. *J. Infect. Dis.* **130**:357-367.
3. **Centers for Disease Control.** 1988. Human ehrlichiosis - United States. *M.M.W.R.* **37**:No.270, 275-277.
4. **Centers for Disease Control.** 1988. Rocky Mountain spotted fever - United States, 1987. *M.M.W.R.* **37**:388-389.
5. **Edwards, M. S., J. E. Jones, D. L. Leass, J. W. Whitmore, J. E. Dawson, and D. B. Fishbein.** 1988. Childhood infection with *Ehrlichia canis* of a closely related organism. *Pediatr. Infect. Dis. J.* **7**:651-654.
6. **Ewing, S. A.** 1969. Canine ehrlichioisis, pp. 331-353, *In* C. A.

Brandly, and C. C. Cornelius (eds.) Advances in veterinary science and comparative medicine, Vol. 13. Academic Press, New York.

7. **Fishbein, D. B., A. Kemp, N. R. Green, J. Dawson, D. H. Fields, and M. Redus.** 1989. Human ehrlichiosis active surveillance in febrile hospitalized patients. *J. Infect. Dis.* **160**:803-809.
8. **Fishbein, D. B., L. A. Sawyer, C. J. Holland, E. B. Hayes, W. Okoroanyanwu, D. Williams, R. K. Sikes, M. Ristic, and J. E. McDade.** 1987. Unexplained febrile illnesses after exposure to ticks: infection with an Ehrlichia? *J. Am. Med. Assoc.* **257**:3100-3104.
9. **Harkess, J. R.** 1989. Ehrlichiosis: a cause of bone marrow hypoplasia in adults. *Am. J. Hematol.* **30**:265-266.
10. **Harkess, J. R., S. A. Ewing, J. M. Crutcher, J. Kudlac, G. McKee, and G. Istre.** 1989. Human ehrlichiosis in Oklahoma. *J. Infect. Dis.* **159**:576-579.
11. **Huxsoll, D. L.** 1976. Canine ehrlichiosis (tropical canine pancytopenia): a review. *Vet. Parasitol.* **2**:49-60.
12. **Maeda, K., N. Markowitz, R. C. Hawley, M. Ristic, D. Cox, and J. E. McDade.** 1987. Human infection with *Ehrlichia canis*, a leukocytic rickettsia. *N. Engl. J. Med.* **316**:853-856.
13. **McDade, J. E., C. C. Shepard, M. A. Redus, V. F. Newhouse, and J. D. Smith.** 1980. Evidence of *Rickettsia prowazekii* infections in the United States. *Am. J. Trop. Med. Hyg.* **29**:277-284.
14. **Pearce, C. J., N. E. Conrad, P. E. Nolan, D. B. Fishbein, and J. E. Dawson.** 1988. Ehrlichiosis: A cause of bone marrow hypoplasia in humans. *Am. J. Hematol.* **28**:53-55.
15. **Petersen, L. R., L. A. Sawyer, D. B. Fishbein, P. W. Kelley, R. J. Thomas, L. A. Magnarelli, M. Redus, and J. E. Dawson.** 1989. An outbreak of ehrlichiosis in members of an army reserve unit exposed to ticks. *J. Infect. Dis.* **159**:562-568.
16. **Ristic, M.** 1986. Pertinent characteristics of leukocytic rickettsiae of humans and animals, pp. 182-187, *In* L. Leive, (ed.) *Microbiology 1986*. American Society for Microbiology, Washington, D.C.
17. **Rohrbach, B. W., J. R. Harkess, S. A. Ewing, J. F. Kudlac, G. L. McKee, and G. R. Istre.** 1987. Human ehrlichiosis, Oklahoma [Abstract 1278], pp. 319. Program and Abstracts of the Twenty-Seventh Interscience Conference on Antimicrobial Agents and Chemotherapy. American Society for Microbiology, Washington, D.C.
18. **Sawyer L. A., D. B. Fishbein, and J. E. McDade.** 1987. Q fever: current concepts. *Rev. Infect. Dis.* **9**:935-946.
19. **Sawyer L. A., D. B. Fishbein, and J. E. McDade.** 1988. Q fever in patients with hepatitis and pneumonia: results of laboratory-based surveillance in the United States [letter]. *J. Infect. Dis.* **58**:497-498.
20. **Tachibana, N.** 1986. Sennetsu fever: the disease, diagnosis, and treatment, pp. 205-208, *In* L. Leive, (ed.) Microbiology - 1986. American Society for Microbiology, Washington, D.C.
21. **Taylor, J. P., T. G. Betz, D. B. Fishbein, M. A. Roberts, J. Dawson, and M. Ristic.** 1988. Serologic evidence of possible human infection with *Ehrlichia*. *J. Infect. Dis.* **158**:217-220.
22. **Taylor, J. P., T. G. Betz, and J. A. Rawlings.** 1986. Epidemiology

of murine typhus in Texas, 1980 through 1984. *J. Am. Med. Assoc.* **255**:2173-2176.

23. **Walker, D. H., J. P. Taylor, J. S. Buie, and C. Dearden.** 1989. Fatal human ehrlichiosis [Abstract D 76], p. 95. Abstracts of the 89th annual meeting of the American Society for Microbiology. American Society for Microbiology, Washington, D.C., 14-18 May, 1989.
24. **Wilfert, C. M., J. N. MacCormack, K. Kleeman, R. N. Philip, E. Austin, V. Dickinson, and L. Turner.** 1984. Epidemiology of Rocky Mountain spotted fever as determined by active surveillance. *J. Infect. Dis.* **150**:469-479.

10. EVOLUTIONARY HISTORY OF CHLAMYDIAE: ANSWERS FOR SOME OLD QUESTIONS, NO ANSWERS FOR SOME NEW ONES

JAMES W. MOULDER, Ph.D.

Abstract

The advances in theoretical and experimental biology of the last 50 years have made it possible to answer many ancient questions about the phylogeny of Chlamydiae, Rickettsiae, Ehrlichiae, and other intracellular bacteria. For example, *Chlamydia* is a bacterium, not a virus; *Ehrlichia* is closely related to *Rickettsia*, but *Coxiella* and *Chlamydia* are not. The finality of these answers and their far-reaching consequences in microbiology and in infectious disease are not generally recognized. However, resolution of relationships among the great groups of intracellular bacteria discloses many questions about the evolutionary history of each group. Some of the as yet unanswered questions about chlamydiae are its relation (if any) to planctomyces, the possibility of extant host-independent relatives, the multiple or single origin vertebrate chlamydiae, and the phylogenetic relations among extant species and biovars.

Introduction

Since the man we honor at this symposium has been a working biologist for close to 50 years, it seems appropriate to look back over the span of his scientific career to assess progress in understanding the evolutionary history of microorganisms in general, chlamydiae in particular, and, whenever appropriate, some of the many microorganisms with which Professor Ristic has worked.

Foundations of Evolutionary Microbiology

The concepts and discoveries essential to reconstructing the evolutionary history of any group of microorganisms are such an integral part of biological thinking that they are often not recognized as discrete accomplishments. Table 1 is a partial list of some historical milestones in biology. You will notice that all these contributions, with the exception of Darwin's, were made after Professor Ristic entered upon his scientific career. He has indeed had the good fortune to live in interesting times.

New Answers to Old Questions

Many long-festering questions about the lineage and interrelationships

J. C. Williams and I. Kakoma (eds.), Ehrlichiosis, 112–124.

TABLE 1. Foundations of evolutionary microbiology.

Darwin, 1859 [5].	Life had but a single origin.
Avery, MacLeod, and McCarty. 1944 [1].	DNA is the genetic substance.
Luria and Delbruck, 1943 [17].	Bacterial genetic systems are homologous to those of other organisms.
Watson and Crick, 1953 [33].	The structure of DNA is consistent with its role as genetic material.
Lwoff, 1957 [18].	Viruses and bacteria are qualitatively different.
Stanier and van Niel, 1962 [9].	Bacteria and higher organisms are qualitatively different.
Zuckerkanl and Pauling, 1965 [40].	The structure of macromolecules changes at predictable rates through evolutionary time.

of *Rickettsia, Ehrlichia, Coxiella,* and *Chlamydia* have recently been answered with such finality that those who have not lived through 50 years of seemingly trivial argument cannot appreciate the magnitude of the accomplishments.

A close phylogenetic relationship of Rickettsia, Ehrlichia, Coxiella and Chlamydia?

The broadest of these old and persistent questions is the closeness of phylogenetic kinship among these and other organisms. The microorganisms in the orders *Rickettsiales* and *Chlamydiales* in Section 9 of *Bergey's Manual of Systematic Bacteriology* [15] were gathered together mainly because they stained gram-negative, could not be grown in the absence of host cells, and were often studied by the same people. The system of classification in Bergey's Section 9 will probably be around for a long time because it provides the framework on which are hung most schemes for the diagnostic identification of these microorganisms. However, it must be realized that this classification is not phylogenetically valid. Every taxon above genus is either patently invalid or highly questionable. For example, from the comparison of 16S RNA sequences made by Weisburg and his associates, *Rickettsia, Coxiella*, and *Chlamydia* are utterly unrelated to each other, that *Rickettsia* and *Coxiella,* now placed in the same tribe, are without immediate relation, and that *Rickettsia* and *Ehrlichia,* which have been assigned to different tribes, are, in fact, closely related [35].

I have two not particularly original suggestions for dealing with these and other related problems until that great day when a complete phylogeny of the obligately intracellular bacteria emerges [see references 27 and 34]. First, regard the present system of classification for what it is, a useful way to pigeonhole a number of phenotypically similar microorganisms, and replace the formal latinized names of the suprageneric taxons--from order down to tribe--with descriptive phrases in the vernacular. This will avoid the appearance of an evolutionary relation where none has been proven or even suggested. Second, completely avoid the use of any formal taxon above the level of genus until that taxon can be defined in phylogenetic terms.

Chlamydiae--bacteria or viruses?

This is a question that never should have been raised. The early giants in the field, Bedson and Meyer, had no doubts as to the bacterial nature of chlamydiae [21], even though the ultimate characterization of virus and bacterium was still decades away. With the truly definitive publications of Lwoff [18] and Stanier and van Niel [29] (Table 1) and the increasingly detailed phenotypic description of chlamydiae [2], there has long been no question that chlamydiae are bacteria. However, the ghost of the psittacosis "virus" still haunts some otherwise respectable textbooks of microbiology and infectious disease. Perhaps the recent demonstration that chlamydiae have unmistakably eubacterial 16S rRNA [36] will finally exorcise the ghost.

A common ancestor for the two chlamydial species?

Although *Chlamydia trachomatis* and *Chlamydia psittaci* share many phenotypic traits down to the molecular level [2], the low degree of hybridization between their DNAs, about 10% [13], has prompted some workers to suggest independent origins for the two species and to ascribe their phenotypic similarities to convergence. These suggestions are made wholly untenable by the findings that the 16S rRNA sequences of *C. trachomatis* and *C. psittaci* differ from each other by only about 5%, while at the same time being deeply separated from all other known eubacterial 16S rRNA sequences [36].

New Ouestions Without Answers

The answer to an old question frequently generates a host of new ones. So it is with chlamydial phylogeny. The new questions are many and difficult. They are so difficult that I would despair of anyone ever answering them were it not for the spectacular successes in reconstructing the phylogeny of procaryotes by examining the fossilized remnants of the past preserved in the macromolecules of extant microorganisms.

The new questions I ask apply specifically to chlamydiae, but, with appropriate modification, they can equally well be asked of any group of intracellular parasites.

Distant relatives of chlamydia?

On the basis of 16S rRNA structure, chlamydiae have no close relatives [35]. However, since it is inconceivable that the chlamydial ancestor could have split off from the base of the eubacterial family tree with all the attributes of its extant descendants, there must have been intermediate forms, both extracellular and intracellular, and there may be present-day microorganisms that share an ancestor, however remote, with chlamydiae.

Weisburg has suggested that chlamydia and members of the genus *Planctomyces* may be remotely, but specifically, related on the basis of the higher order structure of their 16S rDNA molecules [35]. Is planctomyces really a host-independent relative of chlamydia? No one knows for sure, of course, but, among the many dissimilarities, there are some phenotypic resemblances. The most striking is the absence of peptidoglycan, an almost universal constituent of eubacteria, in both *Chlamydia* and *Planctomyces* [7, 14]. Another suggestive similarity is the occurrence of a rare [38] 20-carbon, 3-hydroxy fatty acid in the lipopolysaccharides of both *Planctomyces* and *Chlamydia* [3, 12].

Finally, there is one remote, but completely fascinating morphological resemblance. Figure 1 is a thin-section electron micrograph of *P. staleyi*. The narrow pole of the cell is a holdfast by which *P. staleyi*

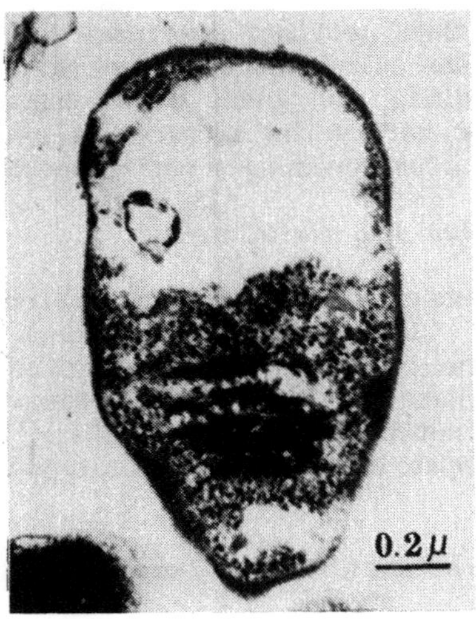

Figure 1. Thin-section electron micrograph of *P. staleyi*. X50,000. From Staley [28].

attaches itself to other organisms in aquatic habitats [28]. Chlamydiae are not supposed to have specific attachment organs. However, there appears to be an exception here. Figure 2 is a thin-section electron micrograph of an elementary body of *C. pneumoniae* attached to a HeLa cell. This is a newly described chlamydial species that causes widespread pneumonia in human populations and has no known reservoir in other animals [9, 10]. Elementary bodies of *C. pneumoniae* are pear-shaped and they almost invariably attach to host cells at the narrow pole [16]. Could it be that these two attachment structures are homologous; that is, do they have a common evolutionary origin?

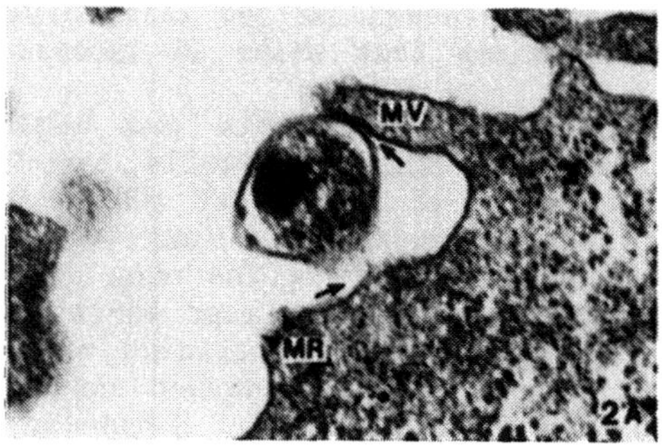

Figure 2. Thin-section electron micrograph of an elementary body of *C. pneumoniae* attached to a HeLa cell. X50,000. From Kuo et al. [16].

Speculation about the relation of *Chlamydia* to *Planctomyces* cannot as yet be taken too seriously. However, if the chlamydial lineage is ever to be reconstructed, then getting some idea of what host-independent ancestors might have been like must be taken seriously indeed, for only then will it be possible to guess what characteristics of extant chlamydiae were present before the extracellular-intracellular jump was made and which evolved afterwards [see reference 22].

Coevolution of chlamydiae and their hosts?

The remaining unanswered questions require knowledge of both chlamydiae and chlamydial hosts. Coevolution of host and parasite is of major concern in studying the relation of ectoparasites to their plant and animal hosts [26]. There has been a long-standing preoccupation with the coevolution of rickettsiae and ticks [19]. However, this concept has been sparingly used to clarify the relations between chlamydiae and their hosts.

The first host for an intracellular chlamydial ancestor?

Microorganisms that may be considered chlamydiae *sensu lato* have been described in coelenterates, molluscs, and arthropods [22]. Figure 3 is an electron micrograph of a cell of the clam *Mercenaria mercenaria* infected with one such an microorganism [11]. All the developmental forms of vertebrate chlamydiae have their counterpart in this electron micrograph. The various isolates from the three invertebrate phyla look

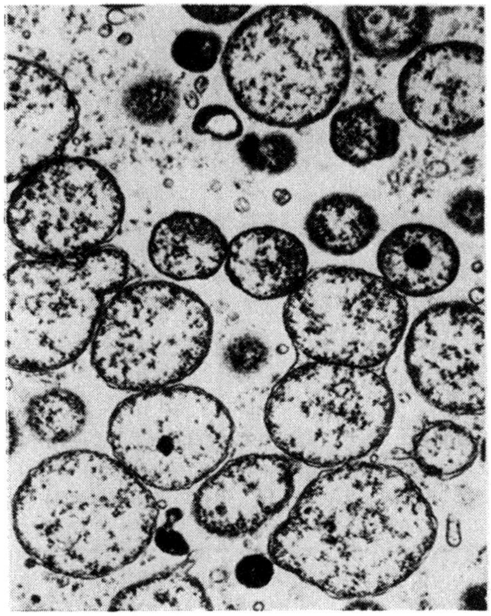

Figure 3. Thin-section electron micrograph of chlamydiae from a *M. mercenaria* inclusion. X28,000. From Harshbarger, Chang, and Otto [11].

so much like each other and so like the well-known chlamydiae of vertebrates that a single breaking of the extracellular-intracellular barrier followed by radiation into the other two phyla is the most likely explanation.

Lower vertebrate hosts for chlamydiae?

Reports of chlamydiae or chlamydiae-like organisms in lower vertebrates have been so rare [24, 39] that they are of no help in filling in the chlamydial host spectrum. Perhaps there is some unknown antipathy between lower vertebrates and chlamydia, or perhaps there are many undescribed chlamydiae of fish, amphibia, and reptiles patiently waiting to be discovered.

Phylogeny of extant chlamydiae?

Bergey's Manual of Systematic Bacteriology divides chlamydia into two species, *C. psittaci* and *C. trachomatis*, the latter being further separated into the biovars mouse, trachoma, and lymphogranuloma venereum [23]. A third species, *C. pneumoniae* has recently been proposed [10]. Because these taxa were established mainly on the basis of phenotype, they may or may not be reliable indicators of chlamydial lineage. So, we come to my last unanswered, or, at best, only partly answered question: what are the evolutionary relations among extant chlamydiae? So little is known about invertebrate- or lower vertebrate-dwelling chlamydiae that this question must be limited to the chlamydiae of birds and mammals, and even here the discussion will not be overburdened with pertinent information.

The idea of coevolution implies that divergence in a parasite population may be caused by divergence in its host population and vice versa [26]. Some, but not all, of the differences among extant chlamydiae may be explained in this way. It will be easier to start with chlamydiae as we know them and to work backward in time toward the first intracellular chlamydial ancestor that I have so precisely located in one of three invertebrate phyla than to work in the opposite direction.

Lineage of C. trachomatis?

It will also be easier to start with *C. trachomatis* than with *C. psittaci* because divergence within this species can be reasonably well-explained in terms of coevolution of host and parasite (Figure 4). Let

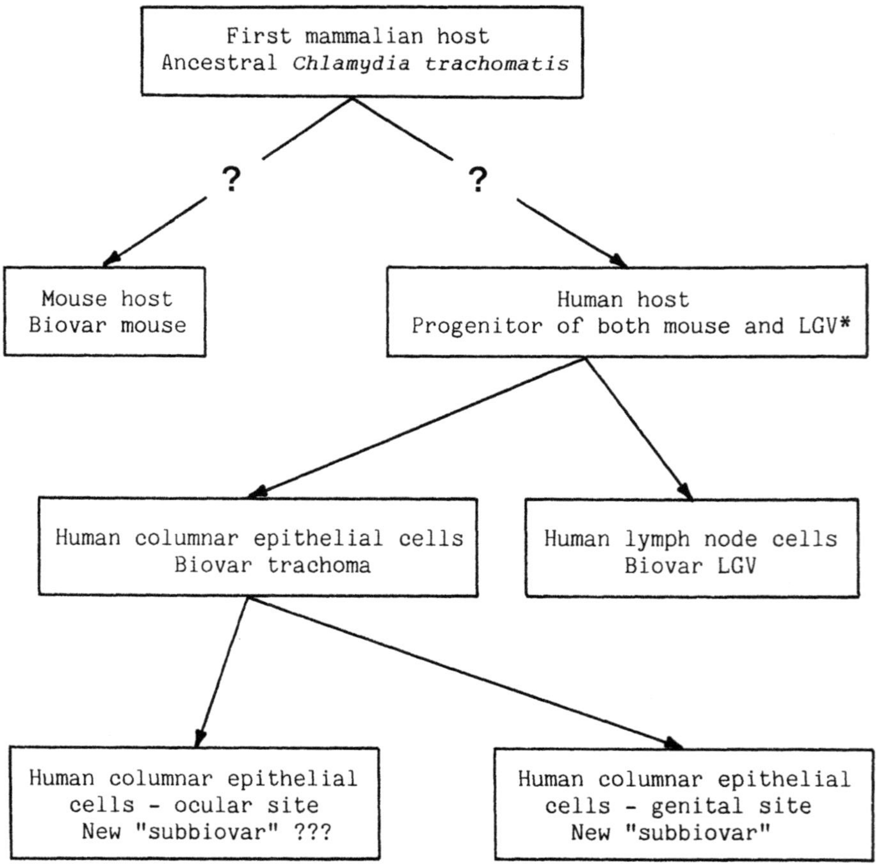

Figure 4. Hypothetical pathways of divergence with *C. trachomatis*. *Lymphogranuloma venereum.

us start with the progenitor of modern *C. trachomatis* living in a primitive mammalian host. As new mammalian species appeared, so also did new chlamydial populations, each better adapted for successfully parasitizing a particular new species than the common ancestor. The mouse biovar could have arisen in this manner. Mice are the only known natural non-human hosts for *C. trachomatis.* Proper search would almost certainly turn up more, but the search might be extremely difficult because the "mammal X" biovars might, like the mouse biovar, be latent in their natural hosts.

The host species, *Homo sapiens*, provides a more complicated problem for *C. trachomatis* evolution--one host species and two chlamydial biovars, each with the human species as its only natural host. This situation may be explained by assuming that the trachoma and lymphogranuloma biovars had a human-dwelling ancestor whose descendants diverged, not on the basis of a preference for hosts, but on the basis of a preference for host cells. The trachoma biovar infects columnar epithelial cells, whereas the lymphogranuloma venereum biovar infects the cells of the lymph nodes [23]. Is this an example of coevolution on the cellular level?

In the trachoma biovar, we have a further example of divergence. Ocular infections and genital infections with this biovar are almost always caused by very similar, but immunologically distinct, chlamydial populations, the former by serovars A - C and the latter by serovars D - K [23]. It thus appears that optimal adaptation to a single cell type situated in different anatomical sites may also require the evolution of different genotypes, which, for want of a better term, might be called "subbiovars."

However fanciful this reconstruction of the *C. trachomatis* lineage may be, it leads to a conclusion that may well apply to intracellular parasites other than chlamydiae. A taxon that appears to be highly homogenous by conventional criteria--biovars trachoma and lymphogranuloma venereum show 100% DNA homology [37]--may show considerable evidence of evolutionary divergence on the basis of its interaction with hosts and host cells.

Lineage of C. psittaci?

The proven host range of *C. trachomatis* is narrow--mice and men--but the host range of *C. psittaci* is almost infinitely broad. So many orders of birds and mammals have been shown to be natural hosts for *C. psittaci* [20] that one begins to suspect that all orders are naturally infected. *C. psittaci* is seldom host-specific [30, 31]. The ability of a single avian isolate to infect other orders of birds, domestic mammals, and humans is well-known. Mammalian isolates are perhaps less non-specific, but *C. psittaci* from one domestic mammal has been known to infect birds, other livestock, and people. *C. psittaci* is also frequently unparticular about the anatomical site and cell type in which it grows, so much so that I will make no attempt to document its intra-host range.

This widespread lack of either host or host-cell specificity on the part of *C. psittaci* rules out a straight-forward application of the concept of coevolution to the unravelling of the evolutionary lineage of this species. It may be that the earliest ancestor or ancestors of modern *C. psittaci* that lived in warm-blooded hosts employed an evolutionary strategy quite different from that of coevolution. Instead of diverging into isolated populations restricted to only one or a very few host species, the primordial *C. psittaci* may have evolved by incorporating into its genome a number of adaptations favoring a wide host and host-cell range. That is, selection may not have been for optimal adaptation to one species but for effective, although not necessarily optimal, adaptation to many.

Such an explanation for the main drift of evolutionary change in *C. psittaci* does not exclude the possibility of the occasional adaptation of a *C. psittaci* population to a single host. This appears to be the best explanation for the evolutionay origin of the recently described *Chlamydia pneumoniae* [9, 10]--long isolation in the human host of a chlamydial population originally derived from *C. psittaci*, so long isolated that a new chlamydial species has emerged. In all seriousness, the pointed-end attachment of *C. pneumoniae* to host cells [16] is more likely to be a late adaptation that facilitates entry into human cells than a homologue of the *Planctomyces* holdfast [28].

TABLE 2. Levels of relatedness among strains of *Chlamydia psittaci*.*

Unlabeled DNA, strain from	% Relatedness to labeled DNA, strains from				
	Parakeet	Sheep	Ferret	Cat	Guinea Pig
Parakeet	100	85	93	37	32
Sheep	82	100	63	37	27
Ferret	100	69	100	24	35
Cat	22	24	21	100	33
Guinea Pig	20	38	25	30	100

*From Cox et al. (4).

A good place to look for host-specific *C. psittaci* populations is in relatively isolated populations of hosts. The koala (*Phascolarctos cinereus*) may be such a host. Its survival is threatened, not only by diminishing habitat, but also by both ocular and genital infection with *C. psittaci*. It is most interesting that recent work has shown that ocular and genital sites are infected by two different strains of *C. psittaci* and that each is distinct from a number of *C. psittaci* strains from other animals [8].

Just because the chlamydial populations now gathered together in the single taxon *C. psittaci* do not exhibit a high degree of host or host-cell specificity does not mean that there is a single freely interbreeding population of this species. On the contrary, by both genetic and epigenetic criteria, *C. psittaci* is a very heterogeneous species. So far only five *C. psittaci* strains have been tested for relatedness by DNA hydribization [4], but even this small number of tests is revealing (Table 2). The cat (feline pneumonitis) and the guinea pig (guinea pig inclusion conjunctivitis) chlamydiae are each not closely related to any of the other four strains, indicating that, despite what I have just said, populations of *C. psittaci* have in the past been isolated enough to diverge significantly from each other. Only the parakeet (6BC), sheep (ovine abortion), and ferret (meningopneumonitis) isolates have a sufficiently high level of DNA relatedness to justify inclusion into a single species, according to recently recommended criteria [34]. Even these very limited data destroy any hope of dividing the taxon into an avian-mammalian dichotomy--the sheep and the ferret strains are more closely related to the single avian strain than to the other two mammalian ones. Immunological typing and DNA restriction endonuclease analysis of a larger number of strains of *C. psittaci* has yielded comparable results [see, for example, 6, 25, 32]. Relatively restricted groups of related isolates have been identified, but broad patterns of relatedness have not emerged.

Perhaps the presently dim outlines of the *C. psittaci* lineage will eventually be revealed as the interplay of the two evolutionary strategies I have proposed. The primary strategy could have been the evolution of genomes with the potential for wide host and host-cell ranges with a secondary strategy of adaptation to and isolation in specific hosts. The host-adapted populations, although isolated enough to allow for continued divergence, would still retain some of the ability of the ancestral *C. psittaci* to infect hosts other than the primary one in which they had evolved. Only rarely, as it appears to have happened with *C. pneumoniae*, would this ability have been completely lost.

Conclusion

I believe the most important general problem in the taxonomy of the obligately intracellular bacteria is reconciliation of traditional phenotypic classifications with new phylogenetic ones. The problem is particularly difficult with the family *Rickettsiaceae*, which, as presently constituted, has no phylogenetic validity, and in the species *Chlamydia psittaci*, which exhibits unmanageable phenotypic and genetic heterogeneity. What is needed to solve the problem is much more data on many more strains. One obstacle to the acquisition of needed data is the difficulty of maintaining and studying organisms that grow only in other living cells. Progress will necessarily be slow.

Literature Cited

1. **Avery, O. T., MacLeod, C., and McCarty, M.** 1944. Studies on the chemical nature of the substance inducing transformation of pneumococcal types. *J. Exp. Med.* **79**:137-157.
2. **Barron, A. L.** (Ed.). 1988. Microbiology of chlamydia, pp. 1-152. CRC Press, Inc. Boca Raton, FL.
3. **Brade, L., Schramek, S., Schade, U., and Brade, H.** 1986. Chemical, biological, and immunological properties of the *Chlamydia psittaci* polysaccharide. *Infect. Immun.* **54**:568-574.

4. **Cox, R. L., Kuo, C.-C., Grayston, J. T., and Campbell, L. A.** 1988. Deoxyribonucleic acid relatedness of *Chlamydia* sp. strain TWAR to *Chlamydia trachomatis* and *Chlamydia psittaci*. *Int. J. Syst. Bacteriol.* **38**:265-268.
5. **Darwin, C.** 1859. On the origin of species by natural selection. John, Murrary, London.
6. **Fukushi, H., and Hirai, K.** 1988. Immunochemical diversity of the major outer membrane protein of avian and mammalian *Chlamydia psittaci*. *J. Clin. Microbiol.* **26**:675-680.
7. **Garrett, A. J., Harrison, M. J., and Manire, G. P.** 1974. A search for the bacterial mucopeptide component muramic acid in *Chlamydia*. *J. Gen. Micobiol.* **80**:315-318.
8. **Girjes, A. A., Hugall, A. F., Timms, P., and Lavin, M. F.** 1988. Distinct forms of *Chlamydia psittaci* associated with disease and infertility in *Phascolarctos cinereus* (koala). *Infect. Immun.* **56**:1897-1900.
9. **Grayston, J. T., Kuo, C.-C.. Wang, S. P., and Altman, J.** 1986. A new *Chlamydia psittaci* strain called TWAR from acute respiratory tract infections. *N. Eng. J. Med.* **315**:161-168.
10. **Grayston, J. T., Kuo, C.-C., Campbell, L. A., and Wang, S. P.** 1988. Proposal to create the *Chlamydia pneumoniae sp. nov.* for *Chlamydia* strain TWAR. *Int. J. Syst. Bact.* **39**:88-90.
11. **Harshbarger, J. C., Chang, S. C., and Otto, S. V.** 1977. Chlamydiae (with phages), mycoplasmas, and rickettsiae in Chesapeake Bay bivalves. Science **196**:666-668.
12. **Kerger, B. D., Mancuso, C. A., Nichols, P. D., White, D. C., Longworthy, T., Sittig, M., Schlesner, H., and Hirsch. P.** 1988. The budding bacteria *Pirelulla* and *Planctomyces*, with atypical 16S rRNA and absence of peptidoglycan and uniquely high proportion of long chain beta-hydroxy fatty acids in the lipopolysaccharide lipid A. *Arch. Microbiol.* **149**:255-260.
13. **Kingsbury, D. T., and Weiss, E.** 1968. Lack of deoxyribonucleic acid homology between species of the genus *Chlamydia*. *J. Bacteriol.* **96**:1421-1423.
14. **Konig, E., Schlesner, H., and Hirsch, P.** 1984. Cell wall studies on budding bacteria of the *Planctomyces/Pasteuria* group and on a *Prosthecomicrobium* sp. *Arch. Microbiol.* **138**:200-205.
15. **Krieg, N. R., and Holt, J. G. (eds.).** 1984. Bergey's manual of systematic bacteriology, vol. 1, pp. 687-739. The Williams & Wilkins Co., Baltimore, MD.
16. **Kuo, C. C., Chi, E. Y., and Grayston, J. T.** 1988. Ultrastructural study of entry of *Chlamydia* strain TWAR into HeLa cells. *Infect. Immun.* **56**:1668-1672.
17. **Luria, S., and Delbruck, M.** 1943. Mutations of bacteria from virus susceptibility to virus resistance. *Genetics* **28**:491-511.
18. **Lwoff, A.** 1957. The concept of virus. *J. Gen. Microbiol.* **17**:239-253.
19. **Marchette, N. J., and Steller, D.** 1982. Ecological relationships and evolution of the rickettsiae, vol. 1, pp. 29-52. CRC Press, Inc., Boca Raton, FL.
20. **Meyer, K. F.** 1967. The host spectrum of the psittacosis-lymphogranuloma venereum agents. *Am. J. Ophthalmol.* **63**:1225-1245.

21. **Moulder, J. W.** 1968. The life and death of the psittacosis virus. *Hosp. Pract.* **3**:35-45.
22. **Moulder, J. W.** 1988. Characteristics of chlamydiae, pp. 3-20, *In* Barron, A. L. (ed.), Microbiology of chlamydiae. CRC Press, Inc., Boca Raton, FL.
23. **Moulder, J. W., Hatch, T. P., Kuo, C. C., Schachter. J., and Storz, J.** 1984. Genus *Chlamydia*, pp. 729-739, *In* Krieg, N. R., and Holt, J. C. (eds.), Bergey's manual of systematic bacteriology, Vol. 1. The Williams and Wilkins Co., Baltimore, MD.
24. **Newcomer, C. E., Anver, M. R., Simmons, J. L., Wilcke. B. W., Jr., and Nace, G. W.** 1982. Spontaneous and experimental infection of *Xenopus laevis* with *Chlamydia psittaci*. *Lab. Anim. Sci.* **32**:680-684.
25. **Perez-Martinez, J. A., and Storz, J.** 1985. Antigenic diversity of *Chlamydia psittaci* of mammalian origin determined by microimmunofluorescence. *Infect. Immun.* **50**:905-910.
26. **Price, P. W.** 1980. Evolutionary biology of parasites. Princeton University Press, Princeton, NJ.
27. **Stackebrandt, E.** 1988. Phylogenetic relationships vs. phenotypic diversity: how to achieve a phylogenetic classification of the eubacteria. *Can. J. Microbiol.* **34**:552-556.
28. **Staley, J. T.** 1973. Budding bacteria of the *Pasteuria-Blastobacter* group. *Can. J. Microbiol.* **19**:609-614.
29. **Stanier, R. Y., and van Niel, C. B.** 1962. The concept of a bacterium. *Arch. Mikrobiol.* **42**:17-35.
30. **Storz, J.** 1971. Chlamydia and chlamydia-induced diseases. Charles C. Thomas, Springfield, IL.
31. **Storz, J.** 1988. Overview of animal diseases induced by chlamydial infections, pp. 168-192, *In* Barron, A. L. (ed.). Microbiology of chlamydia. CRC Press, Inc., Boca Raton, FL.
32. **Timms, P., Eaves, F. W., Girjes, A. A., and Lavin, M. F.** 1988. Comparison of *C. psittaci* isolates by restriction endonuclease and DNA probe analysis. *Infect. Immun.* **56**:287-290.
33. **Watson, J. D., and Crick, F. H. C.** 1953. Molecular structure of nucleic acids. A structure for deoxyribose nucleic acid. *Nature* **171**:737-738.
34. **Wayne, L. G., Brenner, D. J., Colwell, R. R., Grimont, P. A. D., Kandler, O., Kritchevesky, M. I., Moore, L. H., Moore, W. E. C., Murray, R. G. E., Stackebrandt, E., Starr, M. P., and Truper, H. G.** 1987. Report of the ad hoc committee on reconciliation of approaches to bacterial systematics. *Int. J. Syst. Bacteriol.* **37**:463-464.
35. **Weisburg. W. G.** 1989. Polyphyletic origin of bacterial parasites, pp. 1-15, *In* Moulder, J. W. (ed.), Intracellular parasitism. CRC Press, Inc., Boca Raton, FL.
36. **Weisburg, W. G., Hatch, T. P., and Woese, C. R.** 1986. Eubacterial origin of chlamydiae. *J. Bacteriol.* **167**:570-574.
37. **Welss, E., Schramek. G., Wilson. N. N., and Newman, L. W.** 1970. Deoxyribonucleic acid heterogeneity between human and murine strains of *Chlamydia trachomatis*. *Infect. Immun.* **2**:24-28.

38. **Wilkinson, S. G.** 1977. Composition and structure of bacterial lipopolysaccharides, pp. 97-174, *In* Sutherland, I. (ed.), Surface carbohydrates of the prokaryotic cell. Academic Press, London.
39. **Wolke, R. E., Wyand, D. S., and Khairallah, L. H.** 1970. A light and electron microscopic study of the epitheliocytis disease in the guts of the Connecticut striped bass (*Morone saxtalis*) and white perch (*Morone americanus*). *J. Comp. Pathol.* **80**:559-565.
40. **Zuckerkandl, E., and Pauling, L.** 1965. Molecules as documents of evolutionary history. *J. Theor. Biol.* **8**:357-366.

11. RECENT RESEARCH FINDINGS ON COWDRIOSIS[a]

J. D. BEZUIDENHOUT, D.V.Sc.

Abstract

A series of interesting and important research findings on cowdriosis have stimulated and renewed widespread interest in this disease. The most important development is the successful *in-vitro* cultivation of different stocks of the microorganism in bovine endothelial cell and goat neutrophil cultures. *In-vitro* cultivation opens many new avenues of research that should lead, not only to a better understanding of the bacterium, but also to the development of diagnostic methods and practical safe methods of immunization. The identification of new potential tick vectors and non-ruminant hosts, such as the guinea-fowl, scrub hare, and leopard tortoise, emphasizes the complexity of the epidemiology of the disease. Recent isolates of murinotropic stocks of *Cowdria ruminantium* have proved to be very suitable for studying the infectivity of tissue cultures and freeze-dried material, as well as for the screening of new drugs for specific or supportive treatment of heartwater disease. Since there is no cross-protection between various stocks of *C. ruminantium*, the selection of a single stock of the microorganism for the development of a vaccine is unlikely. Although distinct serotypes were found in the genus *Cowdria*, the serological cross-reactions between *C. ruminantium* and certain members of the genus *Ehrlichia* emphasizes the close relationship that exists between these two genera. Serological cross-reactions between the genera also complicate interpretation of epidemiologic data of heartwater disease. The recent world-wide surge of research on *C. ruminantium* will undoubtedly greatly enhance our knowledge of heartwater disease.

Introduction

Research on heartwater disease has progressed relatively slowly as shown by the fact that almost a century has elapsed since the first description of the disease by Louis Trichardt [47] and the demonstration of the etiologic agent by Cowdry [13, 14]. Since then, a further 60 years had to pass before the microorganism, *Cowdria ruminantium,* was cultivated successfully *in vitro* [9, 40]. The lack of progress is an indication of the difficulties that many dedicated scientists encountered during their studies of heartwater disease. Since the first experimental transmission of heartwater disease through blood trans-

[a]Synonymous with heartwater, blacklung, daji enguruti, kabowa, khadar, and magak disease.

J. C. Williams and I. Kakoma (eds.), Ehrlichiosis, 125–135.

fusion by Dixon [15] and Edington [22] and the identification of one of the vectors, ***Amblyomma hebraeum***, research was continually slowed by inherent technical problems. The main obstacles were the lack of suitable methods to diagnose the disease in living animals, to demonstrate specific antibodies in recovered animals, to stabilize the extremely labile microorganism, and to establish *in-vitro* cultivation methods. Further, the lack of a suitable laboratory animal model and an effective chemotherapeutic drug to control the disease in natural or experimental cases slowed progress in finding solutions to the disease problem.

The development of a live blood vaccine helped to control heartwater disease, at least in South Africa. However, this vaccine is far too expensive to produce. Furthermore, the application of the live vaccine is cumbersome and potentially dangerous. A live blood vaccine is also unsuited for routine preventative immunization in countries where potential vectors are present, but where the disease is absent. In such instances, it would be too dangerous to introduce viable microorganisms which may infect, and subsequently be spread by such vectors. The need for a more practical and safer method of immunization is highlighted by the spread of the microorganism to the sub-Saharan Africa and the Caribbean region [51]. The danger of the introduction of heartwater disease onto the American mainland has lead to a considerable increase in research efforts to control the disease by vaccination [59]. This resulted in valuable information becoming available on almost every aspect of the disease. Compared to other diseases of veterinary importance, the recent advances in research on heartwater disease may seem limited, but they are nevertheless substantial contributions to our knowledge. This review will highlight the major accomplishments both published and unpublished on the biology, molecular biology, and immunology of cowdriosis.

In-vitro Cultivation

The *in-vitro* cultivation of *C. ruminantium* in a bovine endothelial cell line [9] and in primary goat neutrophil cultures [39, 40] are regarded as major contributions. These studies formed the basis of more recent studies in which a number of stocks of *C. ruminantium* has been cultivated [5, 33]. Apart from the calf endothelial cell line (E5) originally used, other bovine endothelial cell cultures were also found to support the growth of *C. ruminantium* [67, 30]. Various sources of *C. ruminantium*, such as infected tick suspensions, blood from bacteremic sheep and goats, and infected mouse tissues have been used successfully as inocula in the above mentioned studies with cell cultures. Fresh blood in heparin gave better results than frozen blood. Infected sheep blood which was recently successfully freeze-dried by Dr. J. L. Du Plessis of the Veterinary Research Institute, Onderstepoort [18], was found to be a suitable source of *C. ruminantium* for *in-vitro* cultivation [11].

Morphological Studies On *C. ruminantium*

Our knowledge of the morphology and development of *C. ruminantium* [13, 14, 52] was recently supplemented by a series of papers. More emphasis was placed on the comparative electron microscopic appearance of the microorganism in vertebrate and invertebrate hosts and in *in-vitro* cultures. During these studies, the electron microscopic appearance of *C. ruminantium* was described in the tick vector [4, 37], infected leukocyte cultures [55, 39, 40] and in bovine endothelial cultures [53]. Of special interest is the first demonstration of colonies of the microorganism in the salivary glands of infected *Amblyomma hebraeum* (the bont tick) nymphae [36]. So far, attempts to demonstrate the microorganism microscopically in infected adult ticks have failed. However, salivary gland homogenates prepared from adult ticks were found to be infective when injected intravenously into susceptible sheep (Ball 3 stock) or mice (Welgevonden stock) [7].

The ultrastructural morphology of the different stages and different stocks of *C. ruminantium*, in the vertebrate and invertebrate hosts and in culture systems, are remarkably similar. Reticulate and electron-dense forms with some intermediate forms were described and their close resemblance to the reticulate and elementary bodies of *Chlamydia* have been stressed by many authors [52, 53, 35]. Recently, a new classification for rickettsias was proposed in which it was suggested that there is a very close relationship between *Cowdria and Chlamydia* [56]. This is in agreement with Uilenberg's suggestion that the order Chlamydiales be abolished by reintegrating the *Chlamydia* into the Rickettsiales [58]. In a very recent study, *C. ruminantium* in infected goat brain cortex was recognized by a genus-specific monoclonal antibody directed against the major outer membrane protein of *Chlamydia trachomatis*; this is an indication that *Cowdria* and *Chlamydia* have certain surface epitopes in common [31].

The discovery of serological relationships between *Cowdria* and certain *Ehrlichia* species is an important finding. Cross-serological reactions, of a high or low degree, were demonstrated between antigen from different stocks of *C. ruminantium* and antibodies against *Ehrlichia equi, E. canis, E. bovis, E. ovina, E. phagocytophila*, and an *Ehrlichia species* which is associated with Jembrana disease in Indonesia [38, 24, 19, 12]. However, in the case of *E. sennetsu* and *E. risticii*, there were no cross-reactions [24].

Studies on the developmental cycle of *Cowdria* have not progressed far enough to explain the significance of all the different forms observed in the vertebrate and invertebrate hosts and in *in-vitro* systems. The presence of dense forms with crystalline formations has only been demonstrated in the tick and it is unknown at this stage whether they are part of the developmental cycle [36].

Biochemistry Studies On *C. ruminantium*

In the past, biochemistry studies on *C. ruminantium* were greatly hampered by the lack of a suitable source of purified microorganisms. However, this unfortunate state of affairs will probably change now that the *Cowdria* can be cultivated *in vitro*. The first logical step, namely, the purification of the bacteria from various sources of infected material, has commenced by application of conventional methods of purification such as density gradient centrifugation [48] and lectin cellular affinity chromatography [63]. Antigen obtained through these methods was used to develop an enzyme-linked immunosorbent assay for the detection of specific antibodies in animal sera [65] and *C. ruminantium* antigen in the blood of bacteremic sheep [64]. A Western blot analysis of *C. ruminantium* antigens, derived from goat choroid plexus and bovine endothelial cell cultures, revealed several antigens [34]. Specifically, an immunodominant protein antigen of roughly 32 kDa was identified by goat and mouse antisera [34].

Attempts to construct genomic libraries of certain stocks of *C. ruminantium* were not successful because of a high bovine DNA background [2]. These difficulties have recently been overcome and a pure *Cowdria* DNA library has been constructed [1].

Differences Between Stocks Of *C. ruminantium*

The recognition of marked differences between stocks of *C. ruminantium* with regard to antigenicity, serology, and pathogenicity for vertebrate hosts is perhaps the most surprising recent research finding on cowdriosis. Despite some differences in the pathogenicity of certain stocks of *C. ruminantium* for sheep, they were all cross-protective [61, 62]. Du Plessis and Kümm [20] were the first to isolate a stock of *Cowdria*, highly pathogenic for laboratory mice. This strain exhibited atypical pathogenicity for cattle and it was not cross-protective with the standard Ball 3 stock. Three more murinotropic stocks have been isolated, namely, the Kwanyanga [43], Nonile [41], and Welgevonden stock [17]. All murinotropic stocks of *C. ruminantium* are pathogenic for sheep and goats. The clinical symptomatology may vary slightly from the classical disease and stock to stock variation has been documented. Limited, or the absence of, cross-protection between the strains and with the Ball 3 stock suggest that significant antigenic differences exist between the murinotropic stocks [20, 43, 42, 60].

Very recently, it was demonstrated for the first time that the Ball 3 stock does not offer protection against some stocks of *C. ruminantium*, which are also non-pathogenic for mice such as the Senegalese stock [32], or the Mali stock [21]. These findings emphasize the importance of selecting a suitable stock for immunization which will offer complete protection against all stocks of *C. ruminantium* in the field. These results may also explain the occurrence of sporadic cases of heartwater disease in vaccinated animals. There must, however, be other explanations for the absence of massive outbreaks of heartwater disease in animals that have been vaccinated or were moved from one endemic area to another.

In addition to the above-mentioned differences in immunogenicity between stocks of *C. ruminantium*, the existence of distinct serotypes within the genus of *Cowdria* has now been demonstrated [33]. Applying the fluorescent antibody test, distinct serological differences were shown between immunologically different stocks of *Cowdria* (Senegal, Kumm and Kwanyanga). These findings complicate the serodiagnosis of heartwater disease considerably as it might require the use of more than one antigen.

Significant differences in the susceptibility of some laboratory animals, for different stocks of *C. ruminantium*, have also become evident. For example, it was found that the susceptibility of *Mastomys coucha* for *C. ruminantium* differs greatly from that of white mice (e.g. Balb/c strains). The Kwanyanga, Nonile, and Mali stocks were highly pathogenic for *Mastomys*. However, the Welgevonden and Kumm stocks, which are usually highly pathogenic for white mice, were attenuated for *Mastomys* (5 and 0% mortalities, respectively) [57]. In another study 60% mortality with the Welgevonden and 30% mortality with the Kumm stock was obtained when *Mastomys* mice were infected [18]. These differences in results are presently attributed to possible genetic differences between strains of *Mastomys* mice. Colonies of *C. ruminantium* are present in brain smears of multimammate mice that die from the Kwanyanga and Mali stocks. Although *Mastomys* were infrequently killed by the Welgevonden and Kumm stocks, the surviving mice were shown to be carriers of the microorganism [57]. A variation in the susceptibility of certain strains of laboratory mice for the Kwanyanga stock was described previously [46]. The disease in laboratory animals is complicated by a variation in the pathogenicity of different stocks of *C. ruminantium*, susceptibility of strains of laboratory animals, and differences in pathogenicity of some stocks according to the route of infection [42]. Resistance to heartwater disease in Guadeloupean goats may be due to a recessive sex-linked gene [45]. Therefore, breeding of heartwater-resistant animals may be possible. This could have a tremendous impact on the control of the disease, especially in countries where the vaccination of animals is sometimes problematic due to a lack of suitable facilities or infrastructure.

Studies On The Transmission Of *C. ruminantium*

Amblyomma ticks acquire an infection by *C. ruminantium* through feeding on bacteremic hosts either reinfected immune or subclinically infected [6]. Therefore, heartwater disease may be maintained in the absence of a wild reservoir host [47]. During recent studies on the acquisition of the infection by ticks, it was established that the blood of bacteremic goats and sheep is infective for ticks for only a limited period of 8 days, which includes the febrile reaction after a primary infection [3, 7]. Goats recovering from heartwater disease may not be reservoirs of *C. ruminantium*, with one exception out of 16 [3]. The infection rate of ticks in the field is very low, usually below 1-7% [17, 12]. However, it is doubtful whether ticks will only become infected while feeding on bacteremic hosts, since in heartwater disease endemic areas, there are usually very few clinically affected animals. Furthermore, if the blood of cattle is only infective for a limited period, as is the case in sheep and goats, then there are bound to be other ways by which ticks can become infected.

Transovarial transmission was proved experimentally [8]. However, transmission was very limited and much more work is needed before this mechanism can be incriminated as the main route. The fact that *C. ruminantium* is sometimes present in the salivary glands [36] or hemolymph [17], is an indication that some ticks develop a generalized infection, which greatly increases the chances for transovarial transmission of tick-borne rickettsias [10]. The conditions required for the development of a possible generalized infection in the tick are unknown at this stage and must be investigated. The feeding of field-collected *Amblyomma* larvae on susceptible animals is another way in which the possible occurrence of transovarial transmission of *C. ruminantium* could be established.

The close relationship that exists between *Amblyomma* ticks and reptiles [25], and between *C. ruminantium* and *Amblyomma* ticks stimulated investigations into the vector potential of the leopard tortoise, *Geochelone pardalis*, which is a known host for *A. hebraeum* nymphae [66, 16]. Subsequently, the leopard tortoise was shown to be a sub-clinical carrier of *C. ruminantium* (Ball 3 stock) and *A. hebraeum* nymphae were infected by feeding on bacteremic animals. Also, the tortoise tick, *Amblyomma marmoreum*, is a suitable experimental vector of heartwater disease because it became infected while feeding on bacteremic tortoises and sheep [7]. Similar studies with the crowned guinea fowl, *Numida meleagris*, and scrub hare, *Lepus saxitilis*, proved that these animals are also potential hosts for *C. ruminantium*. Both these animals are very good hosts for the immature stages of *A. hebraeum* [29, 27, 26, 28]. They may play an important role in the maintenance of enzootic stability to heartwater disease. However, field studies need to be conducted to establish the real impact of these findings on the epidemiology of heartwater disease.

Treatment And Control Of Heartwater Disease

Recent research on cowdriosis has laid a better foundation for the development of scientifically sound methods for the control of heartwater disease. The search for antigens which can be used for the development of a safe and practical vaccine is receiving priority in many laboratories. However, it will probably be quite some time before a commercial vaccine becomes available. Some recent work on the treatment and control of heartwater disease, which could assist in bridging this period, is worth mentioning. The discovery of the high efficacy of rifampicin against heartwater is exciting. Equally exciting is the prospect of applying the antibiotic topically (as a pour-on) [49].

Another direction which has received attention is the chemoprophylaxis of heartwater disease. This involves the use of antibiotics in slow-release formulations to control vaccination reactions, or even to prevent natural cases of heartwater. Mare [44] demonstrated that daily *per os* administration of oxytetracycline prevented fatal heartwater disease in vaccinated animals afterwards rendering them immune to the disease. Gruss [23] and Purnell [54] used injectable formulations to develop a prophylactic regime to assist in the introduction of susceptible animals into cowdriosis-endemic areas. This idea was recently advanced by the development of a subcutaneous implant containing doxycycline [50]. This tablet, containing 7.5 mg of doxycycline per kg body mass, was implanted subcutaneously behind the ear, simultaneously with the injection of the live blood vaccine. The slow release of the antibiotic prevented the development of fatal heartwater disease, but allowed the multiplication of the microorganism and the stimulation of an immune response. This method holds great promise for the vaccination of large numbers of domestic or even captured game animals by reducing the manpower requirements. For the correct amount of antibiotic to be administered the body mass of the animals must be determined beforehand. Since a suitable stock of *C. ruminantium* vaccine is not available to give complete protection to all other strains, chemoprophylaxis could possibly be used to assist in the natural immunization of animals against endemic strains. However, natural challenge during the period of protection is of critical importance for an immunity to develop [54].

Prospects

At present, heartwater disease is studied intensively in a number of laboratories world-wide and it is, therefore, anticipated that the increase in knowledge, which is being experienced at present, will continue. The development of a safe and practical method for the immunization of animals in endemic areas and in regions where the disease is absent, but where potential vectors occur, is the ultimate goal. The future looks bright because the material and the methods to obtain such a goal are available. There are, however, a number of other interesting challenges waiting to be studied by scientists interested in heartwater disease and in rickettsiology as a whole. Some studies, such as those on the epidemiology of the disease, can be done independently while others, on the life cycle, biochemical nature, and taxonomic status of *C. ruminantium*, will probably be more efficient if they are undertaken in collaboration with other disciplines, especially with those institutions which are experienced in closely related micro-organisms.

References

1. **Ambrosio, R. E.** Personal correspondence, 1988.
2. **Ambrosio, R. E., J. L. Du Plessis, and J. D. Bezuidenhout.** 1987. The construction of genomic libraries of *Cowdria ruminantium* in an expression vector, gt 11. *Onderstepoort J. Vet. Res.* **54**:255-256.
3. **Barre, N. and E. Camus.** 1987. The reservoir status of goats recovered from heartwater. *Onderstepoort J. Vet. Res.* **54**:435-437.
4. **Bezuidenhout, J. D.** 1984. Demonstration of *Cowdria ruminantium* in *Amblyomma hebraeum* by fluorescent antibody techniques, light and electron microscopy. *Onderstepoort J. Vet. Res.* **51**:213-215.
5. **Bezuidenhout, J. D.** 1987a. The present status of *Cowdria ruminantium* cultivation in cell lines. *Onderstepoort J. Vet. Res.*, **54**:205-210.

6. **Bezuidenhout, J. D.** 1987b. Natural transmission of heartwater. *Onderstepoort J. Vet. Res.* **54**:349-351.
7. **Bezuidenhout, J. D.** 1988. Sekere aspekte van hartwateroordraging, voorkoms van die organisme in bosluise en *in vitro* kweking. DVSc thesis, University of Pretoria, Republic of South Africa.
8. **Bezuidenhout, J. D. and C. J. Jacobsz.** 1986. Proof of transovarial transmission of *Cowdria ruminantium* by *Amblyomma hebraeum*. *Onderstepoort J. Vet. Res.* **53**:31-34.
9. **Bezuidenhout, J. D., C. L. Paterson and B. J. H. Barnard.** 1985. *In vitro* cultivation of *Cowdria ruminantium*. *Onderstepoort J. Vet. Res.* 52:113-120.
10. **Burgdorfer, W., and M. G. R. Varma.** 1967. Transtadial and transovarial development of disease agents in anthropods. *Ann. Rev. Entomol.* **12**:347-376.
11. **Brett, S.** Personal communication, 1988.
12. **Camus, E.** 1987. Contribution a l'etude épidémiologique de la cowdriose (*Cowdria ruminantium*) en Guadeloupe. DSc. Thesis, Universite de Paris-sud, Centre d'Orsay.
13. **Cowdry, E. V.** 1925a. Studies on the aetiology of heartwater. 1. observations of a rickettsia, *Rickettsia ruminantium* (n.sp.) in the tissues of infected animals. *J. Exp. Med.* **42**:231-252.
14. **Cowdry, E. V.** 1925b. Studies on the aetiology of heartwater. 11. *Rickettsia ruminantium* (n.sp.) in the tissues of ticks transmitting the disease. *J. Exp. Med.* **42**:253-274.
15. **Dixon, R. W.** 1898. Heartwater experiments. *Agric. J. Cape. G. H.* **12**:754-762.
16. **Dower, K. M., T. N. Petney and I. G. Horak.** 1988. The developmental success of *Amblyomma hebraeum* and *Amblyomma maroreum* on the leopard tortoise, *Geochelone pardalis*. *Onderstepoort J. Vet. Res.* **55**:11-13.
17. **Du Plessis, J. L.** 1985. A method for determining the *Cowdria ruminantium* infection rate of *Amblyomma hebraeum*: Effects in mice injected with tick homogenates. *Onderstepoort J. Vet. Res.* **52**:55-61.
18. **Du Plessis, J. L.** Unpublished results, 1987.
19. **Du Plessis, J. L., E. Camus, P. T. Oberem, and L. Malan.** 1987. Heartwater serology: some problems with the interpretation of results. *Onderstepoort J. Vet. Res.* **54**:327-329.
20. **Du Plessis, J. L., and A. L. Kumm.** 1971. The passage of *Cowdria ruminantium* in mice. *J. S. Afr. Vet. Med. Assoc.* **42**:217-237.
21. **Du Plessis, J. L., J. L. Olivier, and J. D. Bezuidenhout.** Unpublished data, 1987.
22. **Edington, A.** 1898. Heartwater. *Agric. J. Cape G. H.* **12**:749-754.
23. **Gruss, B.** 1981. A practical approach to the control of heartwater in Angora goat and certain sheep breeds in the Eastern Cape region, pp. 135-136, *In*: Whitehead, G. B. and Gibson, J. D. (eds.). *Proc. Int. Conf. Tick Biol. Control.*, Rhodes University, Grahamstown.
24. **Holland, C. J., L. L. Logan, C. A. Mebus, and M. Ristic.** 1987. The serological relationship between *Cowdria ruminantium* and certain members of the genus *Ehrlichia*. *Onderstepoort J. Vet. Res.* **54**:331.
25. **Hoogstraal, H., and A. Aeschliman.** 1982. Tick-host specificity.

Mitt. Sweiz. Ent. Ges. **55**:5-32.

26. **Horak, I. G., and M. M. Knight.** 1986. A comparison of the tick burdens of wild animals in a nature reserve and on an adjacent farm where tick control is practiced. *J. S. Afr. Vet. Assoc.* **53**:199-203.
27. **Horak, I. G., K. M. de F. McIvor, T. N. Petney, and V. De Vos.** 1987. Some avian and mammalian hosts of *Amblyomma hebraeum* and *Amblyomma marmoreum* (Acari:Ixodidea). *Onderstepoort J. Vet. Res.* **54**:397-403.
28. **Horak, I. G., K. Sheppy, M. M. Knight, and C. L. Beuthin.** 1986. Parasites of domestic and wild animals in South Africa. XXI. Arthropod parasites of vaal ribbok, bontebok and scrub hares in the Western Cape Province. *Onderstepoort J. Vet. Res.* **53**:187-197.
29. **Horak, I. G., and E. J. Williams.** 1986. Parasites of domestic and wild animals in South Africa. XVIII. The crowned guinea fowl (*Numida meleagris*) an important host of immature ixodid ticks. *Onderstepoort J. Vet. Res.* **53**:119-122.
30. **Jongejan, F.** Personal communication, 1988.
31. **Jongejan, F., R. Bax, M. J. M. Meddens, G. Uilenberg, and W. G. V. Quint.** Unpublished results, 1988.
32. **Jongejan, F., G. Uilenberg, F. F. J. Franssen, A. Gueye, and J. Nieuwenhuijs.** 1988. Antigenic differences between stocks of *Cowdria ruminantium*. *Res. Vet. Sci.* **44**:186-189.
33. **Jongejan, F., L. A. Wassink, A. Lillian, Marion, J. C. Thielemans, Nan, M. Perie, and G. Uilenberg.** 1988. Antigenic diversity of *Cowdria ruminantium* and relationship with *Ehrlichia phagocytophila*. *J. Clin. Microbiol.* In Press.
34. **Jongejan, F., M. J. C. Thielemans, and G. Uilenberg.** 1988. Unpublished results.
35. **Kocan, K. M., and J. D. Bezuidenhout.** 1987. Morphology and development of *Cowdria ruminantium* in *Amblyomma* ticks. *Onderstepoort J. Vet. Res.* **54**:177-182.
36. **Kocan, K. M., J. D. Bezuidenhout, and A. Hart.** 1987. Demonstration and ultrastructural features of *Cowdria ruminantium* in midgut epithelial cells and salivary glands of nymphal *Amblyomma hebraeum*. *Onderstepoort J. Vet. Res.* **54**:87-92.
37. **Kocan, K. M., S. P. Morzaria, W. P. Voigt, J. Kiarie, and A. D. Irvin.** 1987. Demonstration of colonies of *Cowdria ruminantium* in midgut epithelial cells of *Amblyomma variegatum*. *Am. J. Vet. Res.* **48**:356-360.
38. **Logan, L. L., C. J. Holland, C. A. Mebus, and M. Ristic.** 1986. Serological relationship between *Cowdria ruminantium* and certain *Ehrlichia* species. *Vet. Rec.* **119**:458-459.
39. **Logan, L. L., J. C. Quintero, T. C. Whyhard, and C. A. Mebus.** 1985. The development of *Cowdria ruminantium* in neutrophils. Abstract 125. *34th Ann. Meet. Am. S. Trop. Med. Hyg.*, Miami, FL.
40. **Logan, L. L., T. C. Whyhard, J. C. Quintero, and C. A. Mebus.** 1987. The development of *Cowdria ruminantium* in neutrophils. *Onderstepoort J. Vet. Res.* **54**:197-204.
41. **MacKenzie, P. K. J., and M. McHardy.** 1984. The culture of *Cowdria ruminantium* in mice. Significant in respect of the epidemiology and control of heartwater. *Prev. Vet. Med.* **2**:227-237.

42. **MacKenzie, P. K. I., and N. McHardy.** 1987. *Cowdria ruminantium* infection in the mouse: A review. *Onderstepoort J. Vet. Res.* **54**:267-269.
43. **MacKenzie, P. K. J., and R. E. van Rooyen.** 1981. The isolation and culture of *Cowdria ruminantium* in albino mice, pp. 47-52, *Proc. Int. Cong. Tick Biol. Cont.* Rhodes University Grahamstown.
44. **Mare, C. J.** 1972. The effect of prolonged oral administration of oxytetracycline on the course of heartwater (*Cowdria ruminantium*) infection in sheep. *Trop. Anim. Hlth. Prod.* **4**:69-74.
45. **Matheron, G., N. Barre, E. Camus, and J. Gogue.** 1987. Genetic resistance of Quadeloupe native goats to heartwater. *Onderstepoort J. Vet. Res.* **54**:337-340.
46. **McHardy, N., and P. K. I. MacKenzie.** 1984. The virulence of two strains of *Cowdria ruminantium* in mice and their use to predict drug activity against heartwater. *Trop. Anim. Hlth. and Prod.* **16**:56-62.
47. **Neitz, W. O.** 1968. Heartwater. *Bull. Off. Int. Epizoot.* **70**:329-336.
48. **Neitz, A. W. H., N. M. J. Vermeulen, and G. J. Viljoen.** 1987. Purification of *Cowdria ruminantium* by density gradient centrifugation. *Onderstepoort J. Vet. Res.* **54**:223-231.
49. **Oberem, P. T.** Personal communication, 1987.
50. **Olivier, J. A.** Personal communication, 1987.
51. **Perreau, P., P. C. Morel, N. Barre, and P. Durand.** 1980. Existence de la cowdriose (heartwater) a Cowdria ruminantium, chez les petits ruminants des Antilles Fransaises (Guadeloupe) et des Mascareignes (la Reunion et Lle Maurice). *Revue Elev. Med. Vet. Pays Trop.* **33**:21-22.
52. **Pienaar, J.G.** 1970. Electron microscopy of *Cowdria (Rickettsia) ruminantium* (Cowdry, 1926) in the endothelial cells of the vertebrate host. *Onderstepoort J. Vet. Res.* **37**:67-78.
53. **Prozesky, L., J. D. Bezuidenhout, and C. L. Paterson.** 1986. Heartwater. An *in vitro* study of the ultrastructure of *Cowdria ruminantium. Onderstepoort J. Vet. Res.* **52**:71-79.
54. **Purnell, R. E.** 1987. Development of a prophylactic regime using Terramycin LA to assist in the introduction of susceptible cattle in heartwater endemic areas of Africa. *Onderstepoort J. Vet. Res.* **54**:509-512.
55. **Sahu, S. P., A. H. Dardiri, and S. H. Wool.** 1983. Observations of *Rickettsia ruminantium* in leucocyte cell cultures from heartwater infected goats, sheep and cattle. *Am. J. Vet. Res.* **44**:1093-1097.
56. **Scott, G. R.** 1987. The taxonomic status of the causative agent of heartwater. *Onderstepoort J. Vet. Res.* **54**:257-260.
57. **Stewart, C. G.** Unpublished results, 1988.
58. **Uilenberg, G.** 1983. Heartwater (*Cowdria ruminantium* infection): current status. *Adv. Vet. Sci. Comp. Med.* **27**:427-480.
59. **Uilenberg, G.** 1986. Highlights in recent research on tick-borne diseases of domestic animals. *J. Parasitol.* **72**:485-491.
60. **Uilenberg, G., E. Camus, and N. Barre.** 1985. Quelques observations sur une souche de *Cowdria ruminantium* isolée en Guadeloupe. *Revue Elev. Med. Vet. Pays Trop.* **38**:34-42.
61. **Uilenberg, G., D. Zivkovic, R. H. Dwinger, A. A. H. M. Ter Huurne,**

and N. M. Perie. 1983. Cross immunity between strains of *Cowdria ruminantium*. *Res. Vet. Sci.* **35**:200-205.
62. **Van Winkelhof, A. J., and G. Uilenberg.** 1981. Heartwater. Cross immunity studies with strains of *Cowdria ruminantium* isolated in West and South Africa. *Trop. Anim. Hlth. Prod.* **13**:160-164.
63. **Vermeulen, N. M. J., A. W. H. Neitz, and G. J. Viljoen.** 1987. Purification of *Cowdria ruminantium* by lectin cellular affinity chromatography. *Onderstepoort J. Vet. Res.* **54**:233-246.
64. **Viljoen, G. J., N. M. J. Vermeulen, and A. W. H. Neitz.** 1987. Theoretical aspects of the enzyme-linked immunosorbent assay technique and its use in the detection of *Cowdria ruminantium* antigen and antibody in reacting animals. *Onderstepoort J. Vet. Res.* **54**:305-312.
65. **Viljoen, G. J., N. M. J. Vermeulen, P. T. Oberem, L. Prozesky, J. A. Verschoor, J. D. Bezuidenhout, J. F. Putterill, L. Visser, and A. W. H. Neitz.** 1985. Isolation of *Cowdria ruminantium* by cellular affinity chromatography and detection by an enzyme-linked immunosorbent assay. *Onderstepoort J. Vet. Res.* **52**:227-232.
66. **Walker, J. B., and K. C. A. Schultz.** 1984. Records of the bont tick, *Amblyomma hebraeum*, from the angulate tortoise, *Chersina angulata* and the leopard tortoise, *Geochelone pardalis*. *Onderstepoort J. Vet. Res.* **51**:171-173.
67. **Yunker, C.** Personal communication, 1987.

12. CURRENT STRATEGIES IN RESEARCH ON EHRLICHIOSIS

MIODRAG RISTIC, D.V.M., Ph.D.

Abstract

Organized research efforts on ehrlichiae started in 1968 when *Ehrlichia canis* was identified as the cause of a fatal disease of hundreds of military working dogs in Vietnam. The advancement of knowledge on the biological properties of *E. canis* led to the recognition of its close antigenic and morphologic relationship with *Rickettsia sennetsu*, the etiologic agent of human sennetsu fever in Western Japan. Hence, *R. sennetsu* was included in the genus *Ehrlichia* under the name of *Ehrlichia sennetsu*. The availability of the latter agent facilitated the identification and isolation of *Ehrlichia risticii*, the causative agent of equine monocytic ehrlichiosis (EME or Potomac horse fever). Accordingly, the current major species of the genus *Ehrlichia* include blood monocytic invaders (i.e., *E. canis*, *E. sennetsu*, and *E. risticii*) and granulocytic invaders (i.e., *E. equi* and *E. phagocytophila*).

Ehrlichiae share many biological, morphological and antigenic properties but also possess unique species-specific biological characteristics. Of the ehrlichial agents, *E. canis* and the disease it causes are the best characterized. The diarrheal syndrome observed in infections caused by *E. risticii* is atypical of rickettsial diseases. Future research efforts should include: 1) further delineation of pathogenic mechanisms; 2) the definition of immunodominant epitopes useful for diagnosis and vaccine development; 3) studies on biochemical pathways and molecular genetics; and 4) search for new members of the genus *Ehrlichia* and potential vectors.

With the exception of *E. canis*, all other species can infect a variety of unnatural hosts under experimental conditions. Recently, however, *E. canis* has been incriminated as a human pathogen based on parasitologic and serologic evidence. Confirmation of these findings await the isolation of *E. canis* or an antigenically related microorganism in putative cases of human ehrlichiosis. The etiologic agent of human ehrlichiosis may be a typical *E. canis* or a closely related variant with a preference for the infection of humans.

Introduction

Until recently, the genus *Ehrlichia* was represented by three major species, *E. canis, E. equi*, and *E. phagocytophila*, the etiologic agents of ehrlichiosis in dogs, horses, and ruminants, respectively (Fig. 1). The advancement of knowledge of biological properties of *E. canis* led, in 1980, to the recognition of its close antigenic and morphological relationship with the human pathogen, *Rickettsia sennetsu* [11, 36]. The other common property of the two agents is their preference for blood

J. C. Williams and I. Kakoma (eds.), Ehrlichiosis, 136–153.

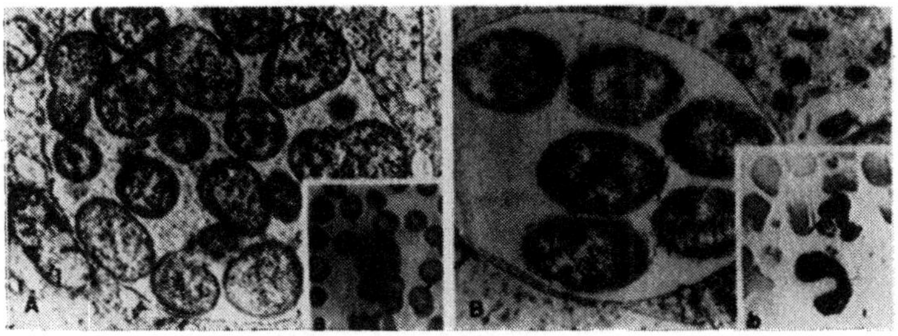

Figure 1. Morphologic appearance of monocytic *Ehrlichia canis* and granulocytic *Ehrlichia equi* (a and b, respectively). Both micro-organisms are enclosed within a cytoplasmic vacuole. Based on electron (x38,000) and light microscopy (inserts x 800), *Ehrlichia canis* form a more tightly packed inclusion than those of *Ehrlichia equi*.

monocytes. Based on these findings, *R. sennetsu* was included in the genus *Ehrlichia* under the name *Ehrlichia sennetsu* [37]. In 1984, the availability of *E. sennetsu* and corresponding serodiagnostic reagents in our laboratory facilitated the identification and isolation of *E. risticii*, the etiologic agent of equine monocytic ehrlichiosis (EME or Potomac horse fever) [12, 13, 14]. Hence, the current genus of *Ehrlichia* includes one human and four major animal pathogens (Table 1).

Human Ehrlichiosis

The first human case of ehrlichiosis caused by an *E. canis*-like microorganism has recently been reported [22]. Retrospective studies [2, 8, 10, 41] based on medical histories, clinical signs and symptoms, hematologic abnormalities, exposure to tick bite, and differential serodiagnosis identified more than 60 additional putative human cases of ehrlichiosis in the U.S. The preliminary diagnosis in the majority of these cases was that of Rocky Mountain spotted fever (RMSF). However, the negative serology to *R. rickettsii* and other pathogens causing similar clinical disease ruled them out as potential etiologic agents. The fourfold rise or fall in serum antibody titers to *E. canis* in these patients, however, provide confirmatory evidence of ehrlichiosis. More recently, simultaneous outbreaks of ehrlichiosis and Lyme disease in members of an Army reserve unit exposed to ticks was reported [29]. Finally, the author and his team recently participated in the study of ehrlichiosis involving an 8-year-old Caucasian girl. Six weeks prior to onset of the disease, the patient was bitten by a tick while hiking with her father in the woods near San Antonio, Texas (May-June 1988). She was admitted into Brook Army Medical Center hospital with signs of recurrent fever, headache, back pain, and general malaise. Hematologically, she experienced leukopenia (1,100/mm^3) and thrombocytopenia (100,00/mm^3). She was initially treated with cyclosporins and sulfa compounds without noticeable improvement. At the time of patency, she was serologically positive for *E. canis* at a titer of 1:40 and negative for *R. rickettsii, Borellia burgdorferi*, and all

TABLE 1. Differential characteristics of species of the genus *Ehrlichia*.

Species and preference	Disease	Experimental hosts	Geographic distribution
<u>Monocytic</u>			
E. canis[a]	Canine ehrlichiosis, tropical canine pancytopenia	Canidae	Worldwide
E. sennetsu[b]	Sennetsu fever	Mouse, dog, monkey	Japan, Malaysia
E. risticii[c]	Equine monocytic ehrlichiosis (Potomac horse fever)	Mouse, dog, monkey, cat	United States, Canada, France
<u>Granulocytic</u>			
E. equi[c]	Equine ehrlichiosis	Donkey, sheep, goat, monkey, dog, cat	United States, Switzerland
E. phagocytophila[d]	Tick-borne fever	Guinea pig, mouse	Britain, Europe

[a] = domestic and wild canidae, Vector = *Rhipicephalus sanguineus*;
[b] = human; [c] = equidae (particularly domestic horse);
[d] = ruminants; Vector = *Ixodes ricinus*.

other potential causative agents. Upon intravenous administration of tetracycline, there was a rapid clinical improvement and her temperature returned to normal. Three weeks after recovery, her anti-*E. canis* antibody titer rose to 1:2560.

Based on the child's medical history, which included exposure to tick bites, typical hematological abnormalities, response to tetracycline therapy and a six-fold rise in titer to *E. canis* after recovery, doctors concluded that she was affected by ehrlichiosis [23].

Unfortunately, in all of these studies, there was no isolation of an ehrlichia from the blood of affected individuals. This may in part be due to the fact that affected individuals were promptly treated with tetracycline compounds which adversely affects an opportunity for successful isolation. Nevertheless, future efforts toward the isolation of the putative ehrlichia from suspected human patients must continue. Once such microorganisms become available by *in-vitro* cultures, they should be properly characterized. Eventually it may be determined as to whether the human isolate is indistinguishable from the prototype canine *E. canis*, a variant that is specifically targeted to human beings, or a unique new species.

Unlike other members of the genus *Ehrlichia* which, experimentally, have been shown to induce infection in a variety of host species, the host spectrum of *E. canis* has been limited to domestic and wild canidae. Recent studies in our laboratory, however, have shown that human monocytes are susceptible to *in-vitro* infection with *E. canis* [16]. Consequently, human infections with *E. canis*-like agents are feasible.

These findings have broadened the impact of ehrlichiae as a genus of great importance to animal health. The recognition of the apparent pathogenicity of ehrlichiae for humans, and the zoonotic potential, places more emphasis on ehrlichiosis as a public health problem.

Etiologic Consideration of Sennetsu Fever and Potomac Horse Fever

For many years the consensus of opinion was that the existence of *E. sennetsu* and sennetsu fever in man were geographically limited to regions of western Japan. The development of methods for *in-vitro* propagation of *E. sennetsu* provided sufficient quantities of antigen for a large-scale seroepidemiologic study [3, 15]. Between 1980 and 1983, more than 3,000 sera from regions of Southeast Asia other than Japan were examined by the indirect immunofluorescent antibody (IFA) test for anti-*E. sennetsu* antibodies. This seroepidemiologic study was conducted as a collaborative research effort between the United States Army Medical Research Unit, Kuala Lumpur, Malaysia, and the College of Veterinary Medicine at the University of Illinois. Approximately one-third of the sera, the majority originating from Malaysian patients with a febrile illness of undetermined etiology, contained *E. sennetsu*-specific antibodies. Thus far, at least three *E. sennetsu*-like agents have been isolated (Fig. 2) from some of the above affected individuals. Isolation was accomplished by way of mouse inoculation and subsequent cultivation in primary canine blood monocytes and a continuous murine macrophage cell line ($P388D_1$). Either *E. sennetsu* or an etiologic agent which shares a dominant antigenic epitope with *E. sennetsu* is present in Malaysia and possibly other regions of Southeast Asia [21].

Sennetsu fever is generally a mild debilitating disease with affected individuals usually spontaneously recovering after 1 or 2 weeks of illness. The symptoms and clinical signs of this disease are somewhat similar to those of infectious mononucleosis. For many years patients affected by sennetsu fever were purportedly suffering from infectious mononucleosis. The Epstein-Barr virus was assumed to be the only etiologic agent of infectious mononucleosis. However, the rickettsial etiology of sennetsu fever was established [24] after the isolation of *E. sennetsu* from an affected patient that was free of antibodies to the Epstein-Barr virus.

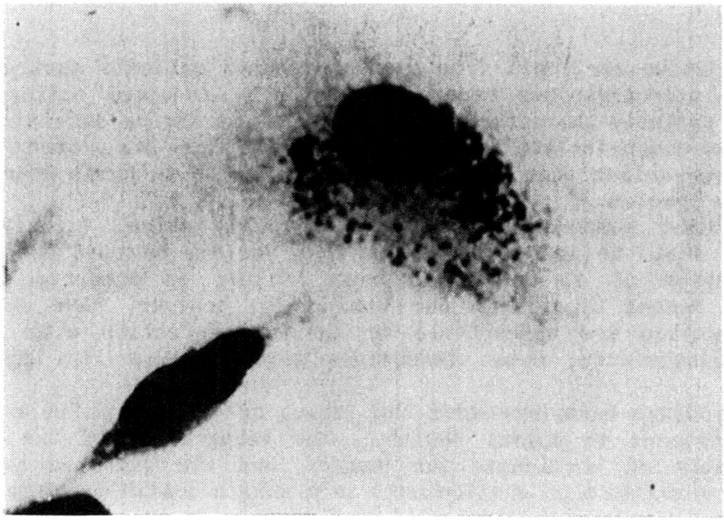

Figure 2. *Ehrlichia sennetsu*-like bacterium in murine macrophage cell culture (P388D1). The microorganism was isolated from the blood of a seropositive Malaysian patient with a febrile illness of undetermined etiology. x1650.

TABLE 2. Seroprevalence of antibodies by IFA test to *Ehrlichia sennetsu* in patients with symptoms of mononucleosis but negative in "monospot" test.

Number patients	Symptoms	Number positive	Titer range
20	Normal controls	1 (5%)	10
98	Infectious mononucleosis[a]	30 (31%)[b]	10-160
8	Hypogamma-globulinemia	0	<10

a = Sore throat, lymphadenopathy, T 101°F, myalgias, and anorexia.
b = Antibodies to *E. sennetsu* more common in patients with symptoms suggestive of infectious mononucleosis than in normal patients.

A recent study in the United States on sera from 98 patients who experienced symptoms of infectious mononucleosis but were negative in the "monospot" test revealed that 30 sera (31%) had anti-*E. sennetsu* antibodies (Table 2). Whether *E. sennetsu* was the etiologic agent of the disease in these patients will require further studies [42].

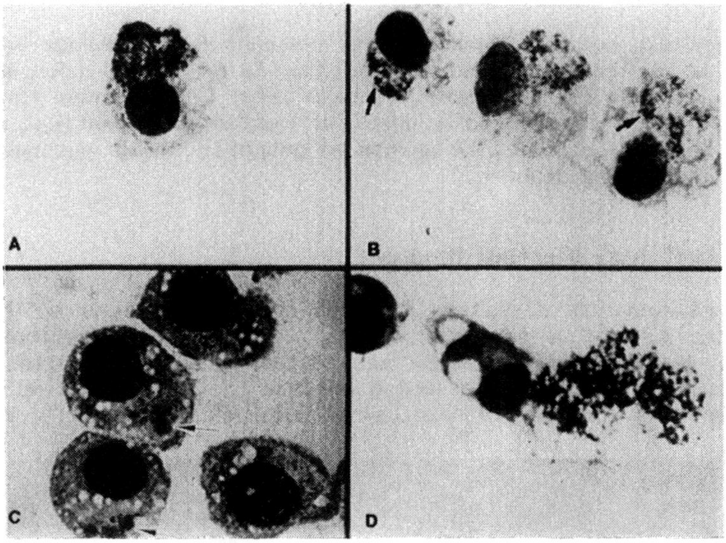

Figure 3. Developmental forms of *Ehrlichia risticii* in the cytoplasm of cultured continuous murine macrophage cell line (P388D1). A) Early stage of development demonstrating a cluster of singly occurring microorganisms; B) Heavily infected cell culture with the development of intermediate cells (arrows); C) Maturation of inclusion into morulae (arrows); D) Disruption of a heavily infected macrophage resulting in the release of the microorganisms into culture medium. x1000.

Ehrlichia risticii (Fig. 3), the etiologic agent of EME, is antigenically very closely related to *E. sennetsu* [12, 13, 14]. Only 5 years ago it was believed that this disease was limited to a small region along the Potomac River in the state of Maryland [20]. Currently, by use of the IFA test [38] and clinical observations, the disease has been identified in more than 38 states of the United States, Canada, France, and possibly, India. Moreover, a retrospective serological study revealed that the disease was present in the United States in the late 1970's [25]. The conclusion is that the disease has been present in the United States for many years. Misdiagnoses were due to a failure of its recognition as a distinct clinical disease entity, the lack of an etiologic agent and, consequently, a specific diagnostic test.

Recent experimental and epidemiologic studies have demonstrated a wide spectrum of hosts susceptible to infection with *E. risticii*. The hosts include non-human primates [44], dogs [40], cats [5], and mice [17]. Moreover, there is evidence that *E. risticii* is capable of crossing the placental barrier. The induction of fetal infection was verified in a pregnant mare that experienced an infection with the agent 4 months earlier [4]. A similar host spectrum holds true for *E. sennetsu* with the exception of cats which, thus far, have not been studied. Very recently, live cultured *E. sennetsu* was inoculated intravenously into two susceptible ponies. Both animals demonstrated a strong serological response to *E. sennetsu* and were clinically protected upon subsequent challenge with *E. risticii* some 100 days later [33]. These findings and other observations point to a need for continued investigations of *E. sennetsu* and *E. risticii*-like agents as potential human pathogens in the United States and elsewhere.

Unique Rickettsial Diarrhea Syndrome

In most rickettsial diseases, the resulting infections by pathogenic rickettsiae are of a systemic nature. In equine infections with *E. risticii*, systemic infection is manifested by variable clinical signs and hematologic abnormalities which precede the appearance of a mild to very severe and frequently "explosive" diarrhea (Fig. 4). Microscopy

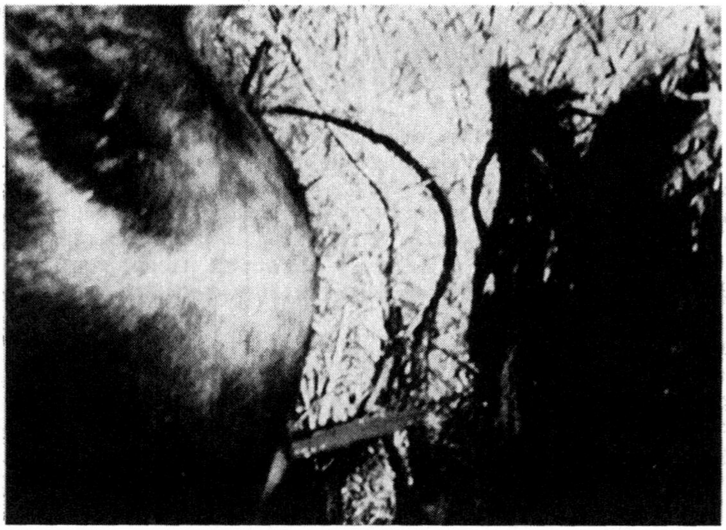

Figure 4. A horse experimentally infected with *Ehrlichia risticii* showing severe diarrhea frequently referred to as "pipestream" diarrhea. Diarrhea is a frequent clinical manifestation of acute equine monocytic ehrlichiosis (EME).

and electronmicroscopy revealed the presence of ehrlichiae in the wall of the large colon and occasionally the small colon, jejunem, and cecum [30, 31]. The microorganisms occurred in the cytoplasm in deep glandular epithelial cells, mast cells, and in macrophages migrating between glandular epithelial cells in the lamina propria and submucosa. The absence of mucosal damage and inflammation suggests that *E. risticii* is not directly responsible for the ensuing diarrhea. The underlying mechanisms may more likely resemble that of *Vibrio cholerae* by the formation of an enterotoxin which induces fluid loss from epithelial cells [7].

Regardless of the true nature of the mechanism of diarrhea caused by an infection with *E. risticii*, the fact that it occurs represents a unique manifestation associated with a disease of rickettsial etiology. Future studies should focus on exploring the nature and cause of this unusual syndrome and determine whether it relates to similar manifestations caused by enteric bacterial agents.

All pathogenic rickettsiae have the potential to be transmitted by arthropods. In the absence of knowledge regarding the nature of the vector responsible for transmission of *E. risticii*, a number of investigators have considered direct contact between susceptible and infected horses as a potential means of transmission. In spite of prolonged housing of infected and control animals together in close confinement, none of the investigators reported evidence of a contact infection. In a recent study, infected tissue culture cells sealed in gelatin capsules were introduced by nasogastric intubation into four susceptible ponies [27]. While two of the ponies developed clinical signs of EME, all four animals demonstrated serologic evidence of infection. The authors concluded that the above findings indicate that *E. risticii* can be orally transmitted, however, the importance of the finding in the epidemiology of the disease is not clear.

Immunopathologic Manifestation in Canine Ehrlichiosis

Canine ehrlichiosis, caused by *E. canis*, is a worldwide disease transmitted by the tick *Rhipicephalus sanguineus*. The disease varies from a mild febrile illness to a severe and often fatal syndrome termed

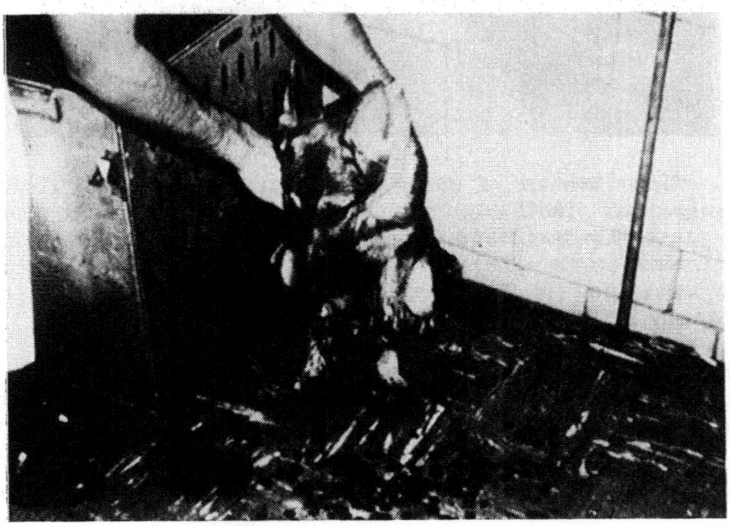

Figure 5. German shepherd dog acutely infected with *Ehrlichia canis* with severe epistaxis. This form of ehrlichiosis is frequently referred to as "tropical canine pancytopenia."

tropical canine pancytopenia (TCP) characterized by pancytopenia, particularly severe thrombocytopenia. The latter is frequently manifested in the appearance of various grades of epistaxis (Fig. 5).

Among various prominent pathological manifestations in fatal canine ehrlichiosis are extensive invasion of organs, with plasmacytes and perivascular cuffing by plasma cells in most parenchymal organs, particularly the lung, meninges, kidneys, and spleen, suggesting an immunopathological etiology. Such an etiology was further substantiated by the finding that lymphocytes of infected dogs exert a cytotoxic effect upon autologous monocytes [18]. This monocytotoxicity was shown to bear a temporal relationship with the disease-associated thrombocytopenia. Further indication that the thrombocytopenia is immunologically mediated was provided by evidence from *in-vitro* studies that sera of *E. canis*-infected dogs induced inhibition of normal platelet migration [18, 19]. Scanning electron microscopy indicated that the platelet migration inhibition factor interfered with platelet migration by inhibiting pseudopod formation (Fig. 6). Affected platelets became rounded and showed evidence of clumping and leakage [19].

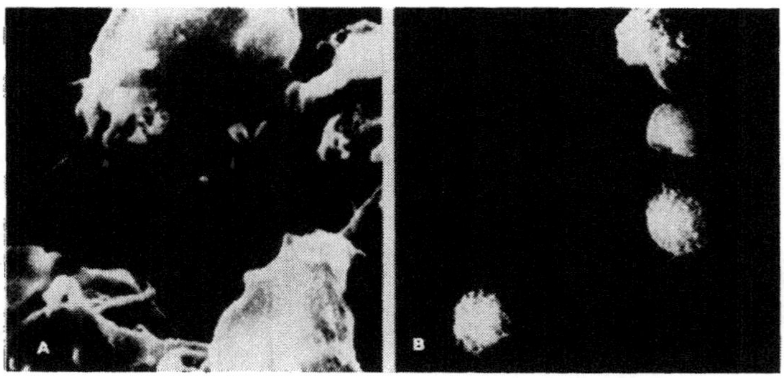

Figure 6. Interference of platelet migration pseudopod formation by platelet migration inhibition factor. a) Scanning electron micrograph of canine platelets incubated in preinfection serum. Note the typical pseudopod formation (x 1250); b) Scanning electron micrograph of canine platelets incubated in the serum of a dog with acute ehrlichiosis. x1000 (courtesy of I. Kakoma).

As a follow-up to these studies, a soluble factor, termed platelet migration inhibition factor (PMIF), was isolated from the serum of dogs with acute ehrlichiosis [1]. The synthesis of PMIF, was found to be lymphocyte-dependent and can be produced *in vitro* using lymphocytes derived from the blood of *E. canis*-infected dogs (Fig. 7). Canine lymphocytes derived from ehrlichia-free dogs can be induced by *E. canis*-infected canine monocytes to produce significant levels of PMIF under *in-vitro* conditions. The concentration of PMIF in the plasma of affected dogs is directly related to the virulence of the infecting *E. canis* isolate (Fig. 8). The PMIF was preliminarily characterized as a heat-stable glycoprotein of 160-190 kDa [1].

Thrombocytopenia, the major hematological manifestation in canine ehrlichiosis, may be immunologically mediated. Hence, canine

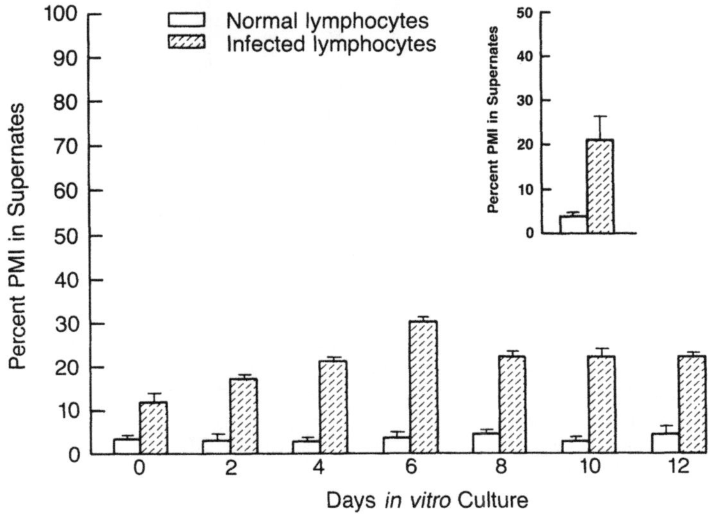

Figure 7. Results of PMIF assay on supernatants derived from lymphocyte cultures prepared from an *Ehrlichia canis* infected dog and normal dogs. Each value represents the mean ± SE of data from three culture supernatants each tested in triplicate. Insert represents average PMIF response in culture supernatants across the entire treatment period.

ehrlichiosis appears to be a potential model for the study of the autoimmune human idiopathic thrombocytopenia and possibly other similar immunological disorders.

Diagnosis of Infections Caused by Ehrlichiae

Diagnosis of acute ehrlichial infections by microscopic detection of the microorganism in the blood is applicable to *E. equi* and *E. phagocytophila* but rarely for the detection of *E. canis*, *E. sennetsu*, and *E. risticii*. Consequently, serologic methods were developed for the specific diagnosis of ehrlichial infections. Serodiagnosis can be achieved with culture derived antigen (Fig. 9). The IFA test developed for *E. canis* [35] was successfully adapted for the diagnosis of infections caused by *E. sennetsu*, *E. equi*, and *E. risticii* (Fig. 10).

The IFA test is applicable to both experimental laboratory and field diagnosis of ehrlichiosis. In dogs experimentally infected with *E. canis*, the period prior to detection of antibodies at a beginning 1:10 serum dilution varies from 8 to 19 days. The analysis of the inoculation data indicates that this variation is apparently due to

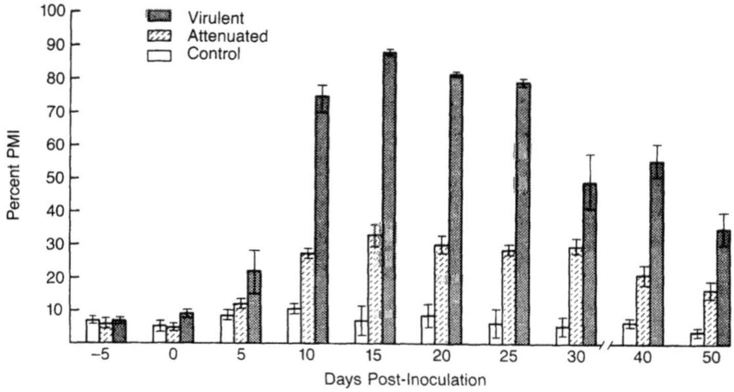

Figure 8. Platelet migration inhibition response in dogs inoculated with two strains of *Ehrlichia canis* in 18- h PMIT. -Virulent strain inoculated dogs - each value represents the mean ± se of data from eight dogs, each tested in triplicate.
-Attenuated strain inoculated dogs - mean ± SE of data from two dogs tested in triplicates.
-Control dog - mean ± SE of data from one dog tested in triplicates.

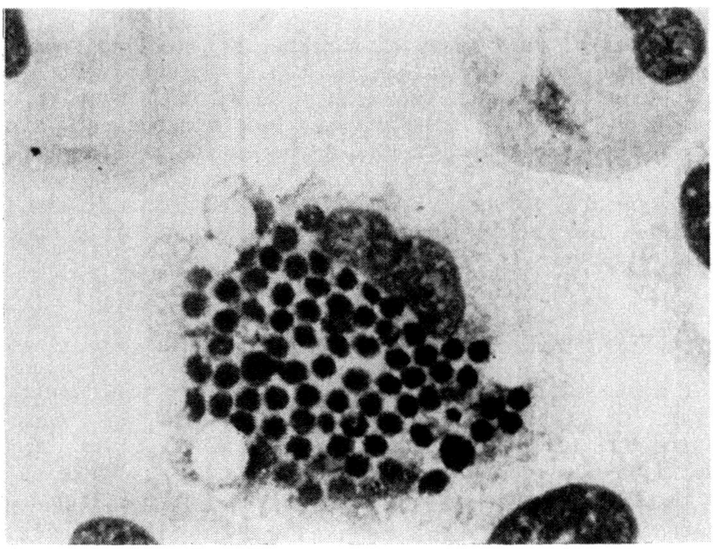

Figure 9. *Ehrlichia canis* in primary blood monocyte culture. In infected dogs the number of cytoplasmic inclusion bodies is usually less than eight. This cultured monocyte contains more than eighty such inclusions. x1280.

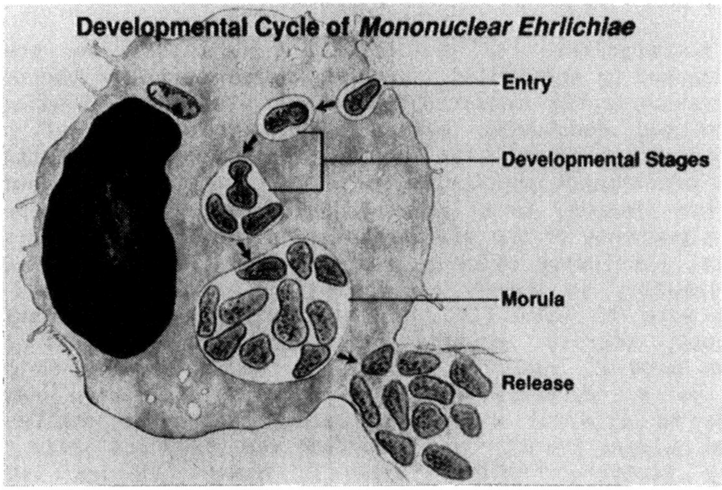

Figure 10. Developmental forms of *Ehrlichia canis* ranging from elementary to initial and morulae stages as depicted in the indirect fluorescent antibody.

individual animal responses rather than to the volume of inoculum. The serum titer in the IFA test may vary from 1:10 to 1:10,240 or greater, depending on the stage of infection, immune involvement of a given dog with the agent, and the breed of the dog. In the acute stage of infection there is generally a spontaneous and rapid increase in titer that usually reaches high levels during early convalescence. Thereafter, the titer is generally maintained at variable levels for long periods of time.

The kinetics of antibody responses to *E. canis* as assayed by the IFA test showed that, at 7 days post-infection, IgM and IgA are the predominating immunoglobulin classes. At 21 days after inoculation, the detectable antibodies are predominantly of the IgG class [47]. Antigens extracted from spleens of infected mice and from infected blood leukocytes have been used for the development of complement fixation tests in the diagnosis of sennetsu fever and tick-borne fever, respectively [43, 45].

Two independent studies introduced an enzyme-linked immunosorbent assay (ELISA) for the detection of antibodies in horses infected with *E. risticii* [6, 29]. In experimentally induced infections, both IFA and ELISA detected specific antibodies before the appearance of clinical signs. The kinetics of IgG and IgM responses as measured by the ELISA revealed that specific IgM was short lived, falling to undetectable levels by day 60 after infection, while IgG persisted for more than 1 year [29]. The authors indicated that the ELISA is more sensitive than IFA test in that the IgM may provide a means for early diagnosis of Potomac horse fever [29].

Protective Immunity in Ehrlichial Diseases

Although tetracyclines [32] are effective antibiotics for treatment of diseases caused by ehrlichiae, there is a great need for the development of immunoprophylactic measures for these diseases. Studies with *E. canis* produced conclusive evidence that the nature of protective immunity is infection-immunity (premunition) with cell-mediated immunity being the predominant protective force [34]. Although not sufficiently studied, the immunity to *E. phagocytophila* seems to also depend on the continuous presence of the microorganism in the host. Contrary to these two agents, conclusive evidence has been provided on the existence of sterile immunity in horses recovered from an experimentally induced infection with *E. equi* [26]. Similarly, although not sufficiently investigated, sterile immunity seems to be operational in equine infections with *E. risticii*. In a series of studies on protective immunity to *E. risticii*, recovery from an infection resulted in resistance to clinical disease following subsequent challenge. All efforts to culture the microorganism from the blood and solid tissues of clinically recovered horses failed. These findings led to the preliminary conclusion that the protective immunity involved in EME is sterile. Based on this premise, the first commercial vaccine against the disease was developed [39].

No information is available regarding the nature of protective immunity in human infections caused by *E. sennetsu*.

Metabolic Properties of Ehrlichiae

Recent metabolism studies on *E. sennetsu* and two isolates of *E. risticii* provided the first biochemical evidence that rickettsia and ehrlichia carry out similar metabolic functions [50]. The two *Ehrlichia* species were demonstrated to resemble rickettsiae in their apparent lack of a glycolytic pathway and in their metabolism of glutamine. In previous studies, *Rickettsia* species were demonstrated to utilize glutamate more rapidly than glutamine [9, 48, 49, 51]. Ehrlichiae utilize glutamate to a much lesser extent than glutamine and glucose was not metabolized [50, 51]. More recent studies showed that the incubation of *Ehrlichia* in the presence of glutamine induces the production of low, but significant, levels of ATP [52].

Conclusion

Ehrlichiae comprise a recently recognized group of rickettsiae of importance to human and veterinary medicine. Their common property of being capable of invading and multiplying within the phagosome of phagocytic cells makes them biologically intriguing. Much knowledge has been gained in relatively limited studies on these agents and the diseases they cause. However, much work remains to be completed to achieve a better understanding of the currently known ehrlichiae and those yet to be discovered. The work of Rikihisa (see Chapter 3) has advanced our knowledge of the ultrastructure of the morphologic forms of

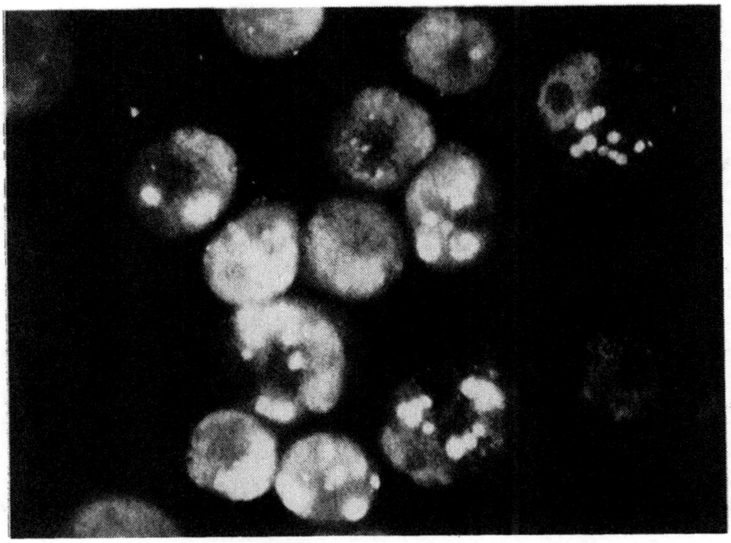

Figure 11. Proposed developmental cycle of *Ehrlichia risticii* in mononuclear leukocytes.

ehrlichiae. A putative developmental cycle (illustrated in figure 11) is indicated by such research findings. Hence, future research efforts in ehrlichiae should be directed to searching for new species, delineation of pathogenic mechanisms, the definition of immunodominant antigenic epitopes of the various morphologic forms and their relevance to diagnosis and vaccine development, the search for disease vectors, and studies on pertinent biochemical pathways and molecular genetics.

References

1. **Abeygunawardena, I. S.** 1988. Kinetics of platelet migration inhibition factor in canine ehrlichiosis: *in vivo* and *in vitro* studies. M.S. Thesis, University of Illinois, Urbana, Illinois.
2. **Centers for Disease Control.** 1988. Human ehrlichiosis - United States, *M.M.W.R.* **37**:275-277.
3. **Cole, A. I., M. Ristic, G. E. Lewis, Jr., and G. Rapmund.** 1985. Continuous propagation of *Ehrlichia sennetsu* in murine macrophage cell cultures. *Am. J. Trop. Med. Hyg.* **34**:774-780.
4. **Dawson, J. E., M. Ristic, C. J. Holland, R. H. Whitlock, and J. Sessions.** 1987. Isolation of *Ehrlichia risticii*, the causative agent of Potomac horse fever from the fetus of an experimentally infected mare. *Vet. Rec.* **121**:232.
5. **Dawson, J. E., I. Abeygunawardena, C. J. Holland, M. Buese, and M. Ristic.** 1988. Susceptibility of cats to infection with *Ehrlichia risticii*, causative agent of equine monocytic ehrlichiosis. *Am. J. Vet. Res.* **49**:2096-2100.
6. **Dutta, S. K., A. C. Myrup, R. M. Rice, M. Robl, and R. C. Hamond.** 1985. Experimental reproduction of Potomac horse fever in horses

with a newly isolated *Ehrlichia* organism. *J. Clin. Microbiol.* **22**:265-269.

7. **Field, M.** 1989. Modes of action of enterotoxins from *Vibrio cholerae* and *Escherichia coli*. Rev. Infect. Dis. **1**:918-926.
8. **Fishbein, D. B., L. A. Sawyer, C. J. Holland, E. B. Hayes, W. Okoroanyanwu, D. Williams, K. Sikes, M. Ristic, and J. E. McDade.** 1987. Unexplained febrile illnesses after exposure to ticks. Infection with an *Ehrlichia*? *J. Am. Med. Assoc.* **257**:3100-3104.
9. **Hahn, F. E., Z. A. Cohn, and F. M. Bozeman.** 1960. Metabolic studies of rickettsiae. Metabolism of glutamine and asparagine in *Rickettsia mooseri*. *J. Bacteriol.* **80**:400-405.
10. **Harkess, J. R.** 1988. Human ehrlichiosis in Oklahoma. *J. Infect. Dis.* **159**:576-579.
11. **Hoilien, C. A., M. Ristic, D. L. Huxsoll, and G. Rapmund.** 1981. *Rickettsia sennetsu* in human blood monocyte cultures: similarities to the growth cycle of *Ehrlichia canis*. *Infect. Immun.* **35**:314-319.
12. **Holland, C. J.** 1986. The etiology of Potomac horse fever. PhD Thesis, University of Illinois, Urbana, Illinois.
13. **Holland, C. J., M. Ristic, A. I. Cole, P. Johnson, G. Baker, and T. Goetz.** 1985a. Isolation, experimental transmission, and characterization of causative agent of Potomac horse fever. *Science* **227**:522-524.
14. **Holland, C. J., F. Weiss, W. Burgdorfer, A. I. Cole, and I. Kakoma.** 1985. *Ehrlichia risticii* sp. nov.: etiological agent of equine monocytic ehrlichiosis (synonym, Potomac horse fever). *Int. J. Syst. Bacteriol.* **35**:524-526.
15. **Holland, C. J., M. Ristic, D. L. Huxsoll, A. I. Cole, and G. Rapmund.** 1985c. Adaptation of *Ehrlichia sennetsu* canine blood monocytes: preliminary structural and serological studies with cell culture-derived *Ehrlichia sennetsu*. *Infect. Immun.* **48**:366-371.
16. **Holland, C. J., I. Kakoma, and M. Ristic.** 1988. *In vitro* susceptibility of human blood monocytes to infection with *Ehrlichia canis*. Manuscript in preparation.
17. **Jenkins, S. J., N. K. Jones, and A. L. Jenny.** 1985. Potomac horse fever agent in mice. *Vet. Rec.* **117**:556-557.
18. **Kakoma, I., C. A. Carson, M. Ristic, D. L. Huxsoll, E. H. Stephenson, and M. B. A. Nyindo.** 1977a. Autologous lymphocyte-mediated cytotoxicity against monocytes in canine ehrlichiosis. *Am. J. Vet. Res.* **38**:1557-1559.
19. **Kakoma, I., C. A. Carson, M. Ristic, E. M. Stephenson, P. K. Hildebrant, and D. L. Huxsoll.** 1987b. Platelet migration inhibition as an indicator of immunologically mediated target cell injury in canine ehrlichiosis. *Infect. Immun.* **20**:242-247.
20. **Knowles, R. C., D. W. Anderson, W. D. Shipley, R. H. Whitlock, B. D. Perry, and J. P. Davidson.** 1983. Acute equine diarrhea syndrome (AEDS): a preliminary report. *Proc. Am. Assoc. Equine Pract.* **29**:353-357.
21. **Lewis, G. E., Jr., A. C. Taylor, D. J. Kelly, A. I. Cole, and M. Ristic.** 1985. Febrile illnesses of man in Malaysia associated with *Ehrlichia sennetsu*-like agents (Abstract). Workshop on

Diseases Caused by Leukocytic Rickettsiae of Man and Animals, July 14-16, 1985, University of Illinois, Urbana-Champaign, IL.

22. **Maeda, K., N. Markowitz, R. C. Hawley, M. Ristic, D. Cox, and J. E. McDade.** 1987. Human infection with *Ehrlichia canis*, a leukocytic rickettsia. *N. Engl. J. Med.* **316**:853-856.

23. **Malpass, D., C. J. Holland, R. A. Howarth, M. Ristic, and N. Rajapakse.** 1988. Human ehrlichiosis in Texas: A case report. Manuscript in preparation.

24. **Misao, T., and Y. Kobayashi.** 1954. Studies on infectious mononucleosis I. Isolation of etiologic agent from blood, bone marrow and lymph node of a patient with infectious mononucleosis by using mice. *Tokyo Iji. Shinshi.* **71**:683-686.

25. **Myhre, B., P. Dilbeck, J. Everman, W. M. Boyly, and C. J. Holland.** 1988. Occurrence of horses positive for *Ehrlichia risticii* antibodies in Washington State in association with an outbreak of foal enteritis. *J. Am. Vet. Med. Assoc.* Submitted for publication.

26. **Nyindo, M. B. A., M. Ristic, G. E. Lewis, Jr., D. L. Huxsoll, and E. H. Stephenson.** 1978. Immune responses of ponies to experimental infection with *Ehrlichia equi*. *Am. J. Vet. Res.* **39**:15-18.

27. **Palmer, J. E., and C. E. Benson.** 1988. Oral transmission of *Ehrlichia risticii* resulting in Potomac horse fever. *Vet. Rec.* **122**:635.

28. **Peterson, L. R., L. A. Sawyer, D. B. Fishbein, P. W. Kelley, R. J. Thomas, L. A. Magnarelli, M. Redus, J. E. Dawson.** 1988. Simultaneous outbreaks of ehrlichiosis and Lyme disease in members of an Army reserve unit exposed to ticks. *J. Infect. Dis.* **159**:562-568.

29. **Pretzman, C. I., Y. Rikihisa, D. Ralph, J. C. Gordon, and S. Bech-Nielsen.** 1987. Enzyme-linked immunosorbent assay for Potomac horse fever disease. *J. Clin. Microbiol.* **25**:31-36.

30. **Rikihisa, Y., and B. Perry.** 1985. Causative ehrlichial organisms in Potomac horse fever. *Infect. Immun.* **49**:513-517.

31. **Rikihisa, Y., B. D. Perry, D. O. Cordes.** 1985. Ultra-structural study of ehrlichial organisms in the large colons of ponies infected with Potomac horse fever. *Infect. Immun.* **49**:505-512.

32. **Rikihisa, Y., and B. Jiang.** 1988. *In vitro* susceptibility of *Ehrlichia risticii* to eight antibiotics. *Antimicrob. Agents Chemother.* **32**:986-991.

33. **Rikihisa, Y., C. Pretzman, G. C. Johnson, S. M. Reed, S. Yamamoto, and F. Andrews.** 1988. Clinical, hystopathological and immunological responses of ponies to *Ehrlichia sennetsu* and subsequently *Ehrlichia risticii* challenge. *Infect. Immun.* **56**:2960-2966.

34. **Ristic, M.** Pertinent characteristics of leukocytic rickettsiae of humans and animals, pp. 182-193, *In*: L. Leive (Ed.), *Microbiology - 1986*. Pub. American Society for Microbiology, Washington, D.C.

35. **Ristic, M., D. L. Huxsoll, R. M. Weisiger, P. K. Hildebrandt, and M. B. A. Nyindo.** 1972. Serological diagnosis of tropical canine pancytopenia by indirect immunofluorescence. *Infect. Immun.* **6**:226-231.

36. **Ristic, M., D. L. Huxsoll, N. Tachibana, and G. Rapmund.** 1981. Evidence of a serologic relationship between *Ehrlichia canis* and *Rickettsia sennetsu*. *Am. J. Trop. Med. Hyg.* **30**:1324-1328.
37. **Ristic, M., and D. L. Huxsoll.** 1984. *Ehrlichieae*. *In* N. R. Krieg and J. G. Holt (Eds.), Bergey's Manual of Systematic Bacteriology, Vol. 1. The Williams and Wilkins Co., Baltimore.
38. **Ristic, M., C. J. Holland, J. E. Dawson, J. Sessions, and J. Palmer.** 1986. Diagnosis of equine monocytic ehrlichiosis (Potomac horse fever) by indirect immunofluorescence. *J. Am. Vet. Med. Assoc.* **189**:39-46.
39. **Ristic, M., C. J. Holland, and T. E. Goetz.** 1987. Evaluation of a vaccine for equine monocytic ehrlichiosis. *In: Proc. Symposium on Potomac horse fever*, May 29, 1987, Louisville, Kentucky, *Vet. Learning System, Inc. Publ.*
40. **Ristic, M., J. E. Dawson, C. J. Holland, and A. L. Jenny.** 1988. Susceptibility of dogs to infection with *Ehrlichia risticii*, causative agent of Potomac horse fever. *Am. J. Vet. Res.* **49**:1497-1500.
41. **Rohrbach, B. W., J. R. Harkess, S. A. Ewing, J. F. Kudlac, G. L. McKee, and G. R. Istre.** 1987. Human ehrlichiosis, Oklahoma (Abstract No. 1278), p. 319. *In*: Program and Abstracts of the 27th Interscience Conference on Antimicrobial Agents and Chemotherapy, American Society for Microbiology, Washington, D.C.
42. **Segreti, J., H. Kessler, A. I. Cole, C. Holland, M. Ristic, and S. Levin.** 1986. Seroprevalence of antibodies to *Ehrlichia sennetsu* in patients with symptoms of mononucleosis. *Clin. Res.* **34**:533a.
43. **Smith, R. D. and M. Ristic.** 1977. Ehrlichiae, pp. 295-328, *In*: J. P. Kreier (Ed), Parasitic Protozoa. Academic Press, Inc. New York, NY.
44. **Stephenson, E. H., A. D. King, J. C. Williams, R. B. Moeller, C. J. Holland, and M. Ristic.** 1985. Pathophysiology of *Ehrlichia sennetsu* and the causative agent of Potomac horse fever in non-human primates (Abstract). Workshop on Diseases Caused by Leukocytic Rickettsiae of Man and Animals, July 14-16, 1985. University of Illinois, Urbana, Champaign, IL.
45. **Tachibana, N., T. Kusaba, I. Matsumoto, and Y. Kobayashi.** 1975. Purification of complement-fixing antigen of *Rickettsia sennetsu* by ether treatment. *Infect. Immun.* **13**:1030-1036.
46. **Taylor, J. P., T. G. Betz, D. B. Fishbein, M. A. Roberts, J. Dawson, and M. Ristic.** 1988. Serologic evidence of possible human infection with *Ehrlichia*. *J. Infect. Dis.* **158**:217-220.
47. **Weisiger, R. M., M. Ristic, and D. L. Huxsoll.** 1975. Kinetics of antibody response to *Ehrlichia canis* assayed by the indirect fluorescent antibody method. *Am. J. Vet. Res.* **36**:689-694.
48. **Weiss, E.** 1973. Growth and physiology of rickettsiae. *Bacteriol. Rev.* **37**:259-283.
49. **Weiss, E.** 1982. The biology of rickettsiae. *Ann. Rev. Microbiol.* **36**:345-370.
50. **Weiss, E., G. A. Dasch, Y. H. Kang, and H. N. Westfall.** 1988. Substrate utilization by *Ehrlichia sennetsu* and *Ehrlichia risticii* separated from host constituents by Renografin gradient centrifugation. *J. Bacteriol.* **170**:5012-5017.

51. **Weiss, E., H. B. Rees, Jr, and J. R. Hayes.** 1967. Metabolic activity of purified suspensions of *Rickettsia rickettsii*. *Nature* (London), **213**:1020-1022.
52. **Weiss, E., J. C. Williams, G. A. Dasch, and Y-H. Kang.** 1989. Energy metabolism of monocytic *Ehrlichia*. *Proc. Natl. Acad. Sci. USA*. **86**:1674-1678.

13. EPILOGUE

J. C. Williams, Ph.D.
I. Kakoma, D.V.M., Ph.D.

The integrated presentations of this book constitute the research progress and problems encountered in the study of diseases caused by members of the genus *Ehrlichia* of the family Rickettsiaceae. The contributions describe the recognition of ehrlichiosis, in particular, and rickettsioses, in general, as human and animal diseases with worldwide distribution. Intensive scientific research has identified ehrlichiae as significant intracellular bacterial pathogens of leukocytes. Human ehrlichiosis, a disease purportedly caused by the leukocytic ehrlichiae [6], is among the newly recognized diseases, namely, acquired immunodeficiency syndrome caused by human immunodeficiency virus [5], Legionnaires' disease caused by *Legionella species* [7], and Lyme disease caused by *Borrelia burgdorferi* [1].

The growth of the obligate intracellular bacterial pathogens in specific compartments of the eukaryotes is obviously a mechanism for the evasion of the immune response of the host [15]. Members of the genera *Ehrlichia, Cowdria*, and *Chlamydia* grow in the eukaryote phagosome; whereas, members of the genera *Rickettsia* and *Coxiella* grow in the eukaryote cytoplasm and phagolysosome, respectively. This compartmentalized specificity for growth within the eukaryote is an important factor in the biology of the microorganisms (Chapter 5).

Ultrastructural analyses of the various microorganisms indicate that they are significantly different (Chapter 3). Furthermore, the heterogeneity of the cell-types within each genus, except for *Rickettsia*, suggests a complex developmental cycle, which consists of small and large pleomorphic forms (Chapter 3 and 12). The observed ultrastructural differences between the cell types of the ehrlichiae may reflect changes in the antigenic structure of the cell wall. Recent studies of the antigenic structure of *C. burnetii* clearly showed that the observed ultrastructural differences between the cell types reflected different cell-associated antigens [14]. Such antigenic shifts are important considerations for the design of diagnostic reagents and the development of efficacious vaccines.

Our knowledge of the genetic and antigenic relatedness of the ehrlichiae to other obligate intracellular bacteria is incomplete. We know that attempts to classify microorganisms according to the site of replication within the eukaryote is a very poor taxonomic characteristic (Chapters 4 and 10). Although much taxonomic information has been collated (Chapters 4, 10, and 11), more research is required to establish the true relationships between these obligate intracellular pathogens.

Ehrlichiosis, first recognized from studies of diseases of veterinary importance, is a tick-transmitted disease of wild and domestic animals. Epizootiologic information indicates that ehrlichiae are

J. C. Williams and I. Kakoma (eds.), Ehrlichiosis, 154–158.

primarily parasites of arthropods that incidentally infect vertebrates, especially canidae, equidae and bovidae hosts. The recent recognition that ehrlichiosis occurs in humans strongly suggests that the disease may be a zoonosis. The zoonotic potential is further strengthened by the ability of ehrlichiae to infect nonhuman primates (Chapter 8). The infection of humans and a variety of wild and domesticated animals by ehrlichiae causes insidious diseases, which generally go unrecognized by physicians and veterinarians. The severity of the disease in humans and animals may vary depending on the genetics and immune competence of the host, and, perhaps, the strain of ehrlichia causing the infection.

The pathogenesis of ehrlichiosis is still obscure, although a variety of hematopoietic and immune-related dysfunctions have been recognized (Chapter 1, 7 and 12). The nonspecific clinical signs of human ehrlichiosis (Chapter 9), canine ehrlichiosis (Chapters 1 and 7), and equine monocytic ehrlichiosis (EME) (Chapter 6) require the consideration of several diseases to obtain a differential diagnosis. The presumptive diagnosis of ehrlichiosis can be achieved either by demonstration of typical intraleukocytic (i.e., morula) inclusions or a high antibody titer to the putative etiologic microorganism. Inclusions are rarely observed due to the low level of ehrlichemia in most cases. For the diagnosis of ehrlichiosis caused by either *E. sennetus*, *E. canis*, or *E. risticii*, whole bacterial antigens are produced by *in-vitro* cultivation and used in the indirect immunofluorescent antibody (IFA) test (Chapter 2). In general, the detection of a fourfold rise or fall of specific antibody is diagnostic for ehrlichiosis. However, the clinical picture must be consistent with the serologic data and pertinent epidemiologic information. Although the IFA test is widely used, an enzyme-linked immunosorbent assay (ELISA) has been developed for the detection of antibodies against *E. risticii* [3, 9]. Also, a dot-enzyme immuno-assay (DOT-EIA) has been developed for the detection of specific antibody (Ma, S. J., *et al.*, unpublished data). More specific diagnostic tests for the detection of antibodies, antigens, and nucleic acids are under development.

What does a positive titer by the IFA test for EME really mean in the diagnosis of the disease? Recently, Goetz *et al.* [4] used the IFA test for EME to measure the seroprevalence of the disease among 1,367 horses in Illinois. They concluded that nearly 60% of the seropositive horses had not been clinically ill and that exposure to *E. risticii* is common. In most cases EME was obviously subclinical and the agent was cleared spontaneously without leaving a carrier state. The authors concluded that EME appears to be less severe than previously believed [11] and it was self-limiting [4]. We now know that seropositivity is a presumptive diagnosis of EME which must be further supported by the clinical syndrome and appropriate differential diagnostic criteria. The incidence and severity of chronic disease after the initial stages of EME are unknown.

There is a need to develop immunoprophylactic measures for the prevention and control of ehrlichial diseases. An effective vaccine against EME has been developed [12]. The EME vaccine appears to be efficacious, but problems of prolonged cell-mediated immunity still remain. Although clinical disease may be managed by secondary chemoprophylaxis with tetracycline, vaccination remains the preferred means for the prevention of disease.

Canine ehrlichiosis is the best-studied animal model (Chapter 1 and 12). Experimental laboratory studies have revealed that the breed of the dog is critical for the investigation of early, intermediate and late stages of the disease. Although Beagle and German shepherd dogs have been used experimentally, other breeds may show significant variations in severity of canine ehrlichiosis. In the German shepherd dog, hematopoietic insufficiency is a hallmark of the chronic phase, which is often fatal after the disease progresses to the aplastic anemia stage (Chapter 1). The disease course in German shepherd dogs is possibly accelerated by either stem-cell or microenvironment injury. The preferential infection of mononuclear cells required for cellular-immune responses may alter cell-membrane antigens and facilitate either humoral or cellular autoimmune reactions. An immune mechanism in the pathogenesis of aplastic anemia has been suggested by the observation that specific and nonspecific immunosuppression is induced after the infection of German shepherd dogs with *E. canis* [8]. These findings suggest that persistent aplasia may be the result of i) preferential infection of stem cells or ii) autoimmune-mediated elimination of stem cells and the microenvironment. In the former pathogenic mechanism, one would predict that antibiotic treatment followed by bone marrow transplantation would promote hematopoietic recovery, while the latter pathogenic mechanism would preclude hematopoiesis by immune elimination of the transplant. To our knowledge, these experiments have not been performed in experimental canine ehrlichiosis.

Diagnosis of human ehrlichiosis suggests that ehrlichiae are successfully transmitted to humans by an, as yet, undefined mechanism. The ehrlichiae were undoubtedly well established in the environment before they were recognized as human pathogens. The zoonotic potential of human ehrlichiosis is clearly indicated by the high proportion of cases with a history of recent tick exposure (Chapter 9). The differential diagnosis of human ehrlichiosis requires the consideration of at least six tick-borne and six other diseases (Chapter 9, Table 4). Noteworthy among the laboratory findings is the suggestion of hematologic abnormalities associated with human ehrlichiosis (Chapter 9, Tables 2 and 3). Although most patients had normal bone marrow histology, a few had hypoplasia, which suggests that the human *E. canis*-like agent induced the suppression of the bone marrow. Infection of humans by *E. sennetsu* results in an acute febrile illness with lymphocytosis and postauricular and posterior cervical lymphadenopathy similar to infectious mononucleosis (Chapters 1 and 12)[10]. The propensity of the purported *E. canis*-like microorganism to induce disease in humans indicates the need for seroepidemiology studies to determine the incidence of ehrlichiosis among individuals with aplastic anemia [2, 16], infectious mononucleosis [13], other chronic diseases, and miscellaneous fevers of unknown etiology.

References

1. **Burgdorfer, W., A. G. Barbour, S. F. Hayes, J. L. Benach, E. Grunwaldt, and J. P. Davis.** 1982. Lyme disease - a tick-borne

spirochetosis? *Science* **216**:1317-1319.

2. **Camitta, B. M., R. Storb, and E. D. Thomas.** 1982. Aplastic anemia: pathogenesis, diagnosis, treatment, and prognosis. *N. Engl. J. Med.* **306**:645-652.
3. **Dutta, S. K., Ac. C. Myrup, R. M. Rice, M. G. Robl, and R. C. Hammond.** 1985. Experimental reproduction of Potomac horse fever in horses with a newly isolated *Ehrlichia* organism. *J. Clin. Microbiol.* **22**:265-269.
4. **Goetz, T. E., C. J. Holland, J. E. Dawson, M. Ristic, K. Skibbe, K. C. Deegan, P. J. Johnson, D. J. Schaeffer, and G. J. Baker.** 1989. Monthly prevalence (1986) of antibody titers against equine monocytic ehrlichiosis in apparently healthy horses in Illinois. *Am. J. Vet. Res.* **50**:1936-1939.
5. **Ho, D. D., R. J. Pomerantz, and J. C. Kaplan.** 1987. Pathogenesis of infection with human immunodeficiency virus. *N. Engl. J. Med.* **317**:278-286.
6. **Maeda, K., N. Markowitz, R. C. Hawley, M. Ristic, D. Cox, and J. E. McDade.** 1987. Human infection with *Ehrlichia canis*, a leukocytic rickettsia. *N. Engl. J. Med.* **316**:853-856.
7. **McDade, J. E., C. C. Shepard, D. W. Fraser, T. F. Tsai, M. A. Redus, W. R. Dowdle, and the Laboratory Investigation Team.** 1977. Legionnaires' disease: Isolation of a bacterium and demonstration of its role in other respiratory disease. *N. Engl. J. Med.* **297**:1197-1203.
8. **Nyindo, M., D. L. Huxsoll, M. Ristic, I. Kakoma, J. L. Brown, C. A. Carson, and E. H. Stephenson.** 1980. Cell-mediated and humoral immune responses of German shepherd dogs and beagles to experimental infection with *Ehrlichia canis*. *Am. J. Vet. Res.* **41**:250-254.
9. **Pretzman, C. I., Y. Rikihisa, D. Ralph, J. C. Gordon, and S. Bech-Nielsen.** 1987. Enzyme-linked immunosorbent assay for Potomac horse fever disease. *J. Clin. Microbiol.* **25**:31-36.
10. **Ristic, M.** 1986. Pertinent characteristics of leukocytic rickettsiae of humans and animals, pp 182-187. In: L. Leive (ed.), Microbiology - 1986. Washington, DC: American Society for Microbiology.
11. **Ristic, M., C. J. Holland, and J. E. Dawson.** 1986. Diagnosis of equine monocytic ehrlichiosis (Potomac horse fever) by indirect immunofluorescence. *J. Am. Vet. Med. Assoc.* **189**:39-46.
12. **Ristic, M., C. J. Holland, and T. E. Goetz.** 1989. Evaluation of a vaccine for equine monocytic ehrlichiosis (Syn. Potomac horse fever), pp 206-214. In: Proceedings, 5th *Int. Cong. Equine Infect. Dis.*
13. **Tanaka, H., and M. Hanaoka.** 1961. Ultrastructure and taxonomy of *Rickettsia sennetsu* (the causative agent of "sennetsu" or infectious mononucleosis in West Japan) as studied with the electron microscope. *Ann. Report. Inst. Virus Res.*, Kyoto Univ. **4**:67-82.
14. **McCaul, T. F., N. Banerjee-Bhatnagar, and J. C. Williams.** 1990. Antigenic differences among *Coxiella burnetii* morphological cell types revealed by post-embedding immunoelectron microscopy and immunoblotting. *Can. J. Microbiol.* (In Press).

15. **Williams, J. C., and M. H. Vodkin.** 1987. Metabolism and genetics of chlamydias and rickettsias. *Onderstepoort J. Vet. Res.* **54**:211-221.
16. **Zoumbos, N. C., P. Gascon, J. Y. Djeu, S. R. Trost, and N. S. Young.** 1985. Circulating activated suppressor T lymphocytes in aplastic anemia. *N. Engl. J. Med.* **312**:257-265.

Index of subjects

Abortions 73
Adenosine 5′-triphosphate (ATP) 59, 60, 61, 62, 65, 148
Aeromonas salmonicida 37
hydrophila 37
Affinity chromatography 87, 128
Agrobacterium tumefaciens 39
Alpha subdivision 39, 41
Alanine aminotransferase 100
Amblyomma hebraeum 126, 127, 129, 130
marmoreum 130
Anaplasmataceae 32, 33
Antigenic characteristics 1, 32, 128, 154
common antigen 46
genus-specific 32, 46
heat shock proteins, HSP 60 32, 33, 46, 47
species-specific antigens (SPA) proteins 41
strain-specific 43
Antigenic variation 36, 42
Aplastic anemia 4, 156
Aspartate aminotransferase 100
Atractyloside 59, 61, 62
Attenuation 13, 146
Autoimmunity 47
Autoimmune human idiopathic thrombocytopenia 81, 145

Baboons (*Papio anubis*) 93, 95
Bartonellaceae 32, 33
Beagle dogs 2, 4, 78, 156
Biovars 22, 117, 118, 119
lymphogranuloma venereum 117
trachoma 117, 118
Blood vaccine 126, 131
Blue-green alga 48
Bone marrow 2, 79, 156
Borrelia burgdorferi 104, 137, 154
lyme disease 137, 154
Bovidae 154
Bovine endothelial cultures 125, 126, 127, 128

Camphylobacter 47
Canidae 154
Canine ehrlichiosis 2, 4, 9, 18, 59, 78, 86, 143, 156
Canine monocyte cultures 12, 13, 15, 16, 17
Caprine endothelial cells 29
Capsular layer 27
Cell-mediated immunity 73, 148, 155
Chaperonin (common antigen) 46
Chemoprophylaxis 130, 131, 155
Chlamydia(e) 11, 13, 14, 16, 26, 27, 39, 40, 47, 65, 66, 112, 115, 127, 154
pneumoniae 115, 120
psittaci 114, 120
6BC (parakeet) 120, 121

feline pneumonitis (cat) 120, 121
ferret (meningopneumonitis 120, 121
inclusion conjunctivitis (guinea pig) 120, 121
ovine abortion (sheep) 120, 121
trachomatis 39, 114
A-C 119
D-K 119
lymphogranuloma venereum 117
trachoma 117, 118
Coevolution 116, 118
Colorado Tick Fever 103
Common antigen (chaperonin)
Cowdria ruminantium 22, 23, 28, 29, 32, 34, 45, 125, 127, 129, 154
Ball 128, 130
Mali 29, 128, 129
Nonile 128, 129
Kumm 23, 29, 128, 129
Kwanyanga 129
Senegal 128
Welgevonden 129
Cowdriosis (Heartwater Disease) 125
Coxiella burnetii 25, 27, 32, 34, 36, 38, 48
Nine Mile 45
Priscilla 45
Crowned guinea fowl 130
Cultivation 9
in vitro 9, 84, 126
in vivo 84
Cyclophosphamide 15
Cytoplasm 11, 13, 22, 27, 39, 41, 154
Cytoecetes phagocytophila 34

Deoxyribonucleic acid (DNA) 32, 35, 39
cloning 32
cosmid 35
genomic libraries 35
lambda 37, 48
plasmid vectors 35
polymerase chain reaction (PCR) 35
Deoxyribonuclease (DNAase)
Dermacentor varibilis 70
Developmental cycle 66, 70, 127
Diarrheal syndrome 68, 136, 142
2,4-Dinitrophenol (DNP) 59, 61, 62
Dohle's inclusion bodies 102
Dot-enzyme immuno-assay (DOT-EIA) 155
Doxcycline 138

Ehrlichemia 4, 97
Ehrlichiosis 1, 10, 68, 100, 101, 106, 136, 154
Ehrlichia (leukocytic rickettsiae) 1, 9, 23, 32, 39, 65, 127, 154
bovis 93, 127
canis 1, 9, 11, 12, 17, 34, 69, 70, 93, 127, 136, 138, 145, 155
equi 18, 69, 127, 136, 138, 145
ovina 127
phagocytophila 18, 45, 127, 136, 138, 145

risticii 10, 17, 18, 22, 23, 24, 25, 27, 34, 38, 40, 48, 68, 69, 70, 127, 136, 138, 141, 145, 155
sennetsu 10, 13, 16, 17, 18, 34, 38, 59, 69, 70, 93, 127, 136, 138, 145, 155
Myayama 59
Ehrlichiae 12, 22, 32, 39
Elementary body 14, 66, 116, 127
Endemic (flea-borne or murine) typhus 100
Endosymbiosis 39
Energy metabolism 59
Enzyme-linked immunosorbent assay (ELISA) 128, 147, 155
Epidemic typhus (*Rickettsia prowazekii*) 1
Ehrlichemia (bacteraemia, bacteremia) 93
Epistaxis 78, 144
Epizootic 2, 10
Epstein-Barr virus 139
Equidae 154
Equine ehrlichiosis 69
Equine monocyte cultures 17, 18, 69
Equine monocytic ehrlichiosis (EME) or 10, 18, 68, 69, 93, 116, 139, 141, 154
Potomac horse fever (PHF) 10, 93, 136, 137
Erythrocytes 33
Evolution 39
coevolution 116, 118

Feline pneumonitis 120
Ficoll Hypaque gradient 85

Gamma subdivision 41
Genomic libraries 35
Gentamicin 70
German shepherd dogs 2, 78, 143, 156
Glucose 16, 59, 65
Glucose-6-phosphate 60, 61, 65
Glutamate 16, 59, 60, 148
Goat neutrophil cultures 125
Glutamine 16, 59, 61, 63, 70, 148
Granulocytic ehrlichiae 18, 136
GroEL 48
GroES 48
Guadeloupean goats 129

Haertwater disease (Cowdriosis) 128
Heat-modifiable proteins 41
Hematopoietic insufficiency 154, 156
Hemorrhage 2, 78
Human ehrlichiosis 106, 109, 136, 137, 154
Human immunodeficiency virus (HIV) 154
Human monocyte cultures 15, 23
Hypergammaglobulinemia 78, 79
Hypersplenism (splenomegaly) 80, 82
Hypoplasia 4, 104, 156

Immunoglobulin 147
IgA 147
IgG 147

IgM 41, 147
Immunoprophylaxis 148, 155
Inclusion 11, 12, 65, 69, 94, 146, 154
Indirect immunofluorescence antibody (IFA) 9, 10, 17, 68, 69, 70, 85, 102, 139, 141, 145, 155
Infectious mononucleosis 16, 139, 140, 156
Intraphagosomal 91

Jembrana disease 127

Koala (*Phascolarctos cinereus*) 120

Legionella bozemanii 37
macdadei 37
Legionnaires' disease 154
Leopard tortoise (*Geochelone pardalis*) 125, 130
Leptospira (leptospirosis) 102
Leukocytes 1, 127
Leukopenia 68, 100, 104, 137
Lyme disease (*Borrelia burgdorferi*) 103, 105, 137
Lymphadenopathy 94, 95
Lymphocyte cultures 85
Lymphogranuloma venereum 117
Lipopolysaccharide 27, 35, 41
Lipoprotein 48
Liver dysfunction 100
Lysosome 22

Macaca fasicularis (rhesus macaques) 93, 94
Macaca mulatta (cynomolgus macaques) 93, 94, 96
Macaca sylvana (inuus) 96
Marrow hypoplasia 80
Marrow microenvironment 4
Mastomys coucha 129
Megakaryocyte 80
Metabolism 59
Mitochondria 47, 48
Monocyte culture 11, 12, 14, 68, 85
Mononucleosis 9, 94
Morphology (ical) 1, 14, 127
Morulae (morula) 11, 13, 25, 60, 69, 96, 97, 141, 147, 154
Murine macrophage cell line $P388D^1$ 17
Myelofibrosis 80
Mycobacterium leprae 46, 47

Neorickettsia helminthoeca 4, 32
Neutrophil 126
Nicotinamide adenine dinucleotide phosphate (NADP) 61
Nonhuman primates 93, 154
Numida meleagris 130

Oxytetracycline 27, 70, 130

Pancytopenia 2, 78, 80, 83, 143
Papio anubis 95
Penicillin 70

Peptidoglycan 22, 27, 29
Percoll 32, 59, 61, 62
Phagosome (phagosomal) 1, 11, 22, 23, 24, 25, 27, 29, 41, 66, 69, 70, 148
Phagosome-lysome fusion (PLF) 26, 66, 70
Phase variation 38
Phospholipase 66
Phylogeny (phylogenetic) 32, 113
    5S RNA 39
    16S RNA 32, 33, 39, 47, 65
    23S RNA 39
Planctomyces staleyi 112, 115
Plasmacytosis 78
Platelet migration inhibition factor (PMIF) 78, 83, 85, 90, 144
    platelet migration inhibition test (PMIT) 23
    platelet-rich plasma (PRP)
    platelet-poor plasma (PPP)
Platelets 4, 78, 80, 83, 85, 91
Pleomorphism 14, 22 24, 27, 68, 69
Poly-beta-hydroxy-butyrate 65
Polymerase chain reaction (PCR) 34
Polymorphonuclear leukocytes 22, 27
Potomac horse fever (PHF) or
    Equine monocytic ehrlichiosis (EME) 1, 17, 22, 23, 68, 73, 93, 136, 137, 139, 141
Proteobacteria 39, 40
Psittacosis 14, 48
Purple eubacteria 39, 41, 47

Q fever 100

Renografin 32, 34, 59, 61, 62
Restriction fragment length polymorphism (RFLP) 34, 35, 49
Rhipicephalus sanguineus 4, 9, 143
Ribosomal RNA (rRNA)
    5S 39
    16S 33
    23S 39
Rickettsia(e) (ceae) 1, 9, 13, 14, 22, 23, 32, 34, 65, 154
Rickettsia 23, 32
    bellii 36, 39
    ionorii 36
    orientalis
        scrub typhus 35
    prowazeki 1, 22, 27, 34
    rickettsii 22, 27, 104, 137
        Rocky Mountain spotted fever (RMSP) 1, 100, 103, 137
    sennetsu (Ehrlichia sennetsu) 1, 9, 136
        sennetsu fever 136
    tsutsugamushi (Gilliam, Karp, Kato) 25, 26, 27, 29, 35, 39, 48
        scrub typhus 22
    typhi 34, 65
        endemic typhus (fleaborne, murine) 100
Rickettsiella 32, 34
Rochalimaea quintana 32, 35, 36, 39
        vinsonii 36
Rifampicin 70, 130

Rheumatoid arthritis 47

Salmon poisoning 4
Scrub hare (*Lepus sxitilis*) 125, 130
Sennetsu fever (ricketsiosis) 15, 69, 139
Septicemia (bacteraemia, bacteremia)
Serovars 22, 119
    A-C, D-K 119
Severe chronic disease 2
Spirochetes 47
Spotless Rocky Mountain spotted fever (SSF) 36, 100
Stem cells 4, 156
Stock (strains) 48, 125, 126, 128
Strain (stocks) 22, 23
Streptomycin 70
Suppression 4, 156
Synechococcus 48

Taxonomy 131, 154
T-cell epitopes 47
Tetracycline 4, 70, 103, 137, 148, 155
Thrombocytopenia 79, 80, 81, 82, 83, 84, 90, 100, 101, 104, 137, 144
Thrombopoiesis 80
Tick-borne fever 10, 34
Ticks
    Amblyomma hebraeum 126, 127, 129, 130
    Dermacentor varibilis 72
Toxicity
Tropical canine pancytopenia (TCP) 2, 9, 18
    Ehrlichia canis 1, 2, 4
Transmission 4, 10, 18, 69, 74, 125, 143
    transplacental 73
    transovarial 4, 129, 130
    transstadial 4
Transverse binary fission 70
Tropical canine pancytopenia (TCP) 78, 143
Tularemia 102
Typhus 1, 4, 36, 39, 100
    endemic 100
    epidemic 1
    flea-borne 100
    sporadic 100

Vaccine 155
    blood 126, 131
    PHF-Vax 73, 74
Vibrio cholerae 142
Virulence 13, 78, 90, 144, 146

Weil-Felix reaction 37
    Proteus OX19 37
        OX2 37
Wolbachia persica 32, 34, 35, 37, 38, 40

Zooanthropozoonotic 100
Zoonosis (zoonotic) 103, 139, 154, 156